Child Language Disability

Volume 3: Hearing Impairment

Edited by

Kay Mogford-Bevan and Jane Sadler

MULTILINGUAL MATTERS LTD
Clevedon • Philadelphia • Adelaide

Library of Congress Cataloging in Publication Data

(Revised for Vol. 3)
Child Language Disability
(V. 2: Multilingual Matters)
Vol.1 contains papers of a conference held Apr. 23, 1988; organized by the
University of Newcastle upon Tyne in association with Sunderland Education
Authority.
Vol. 2 based on a conference held Apr. 21, 1990.
Includes bibliographies and indexes.
Contents: Vol. 1: Implications in an Educational Setting/Edited by Kay Mogford
and Jane Sadler. Vol. 2: Semantic and Pragmatic Difficulties/Edited by Kay
Mogford-Bevan and Jane Sadler. Vol. 3: Hearing Impairment/Edited by Kay
Mogford-Bevan and Jane Sadler.
1. Language disorders in children–Congresses.
I. Mogford-Bevan, Kay. II. Sadler, Jane. III. University of Newcastle upon Tyne,
Dept. of Speech. IV. Sunderland Education Authority. V. Series: Multilingual
Matters (Series)
RJ496.L35C47   1989   618.92′855   89-3177

British Library Cataloguing in Publication Data

A CIP catalogue record for this book is available from the British Library.

ISBN 1-85359-169-6 (hbk)
ISBN 1-85359-168-8 (pbk)

Multilingual Matters Ltd

UK: Frankfurt Lodge, Clevedon Hall, Victoria Road, Clevedon, Avon BS21 7SJ.
USA: 1900 Frost Road, Suite 101, Bristol, PA 19007, USA.
Australia: P.O. Box 6025, 83 Gilles Street, Adelaide, SA 5000, Australia.

Typeset, printed and bound in Great Britain by the Longdunn Press, Bristol.

Contents

Preface

Hearing impairment, whether mild and transient or lifelong and severe can potentially undermine a child's learning because successful communication is at the heart of the educational process.

Changes in policy regarding education of children with hearing loss in the last decade have meant that more children with significant, long-term hearing losses are being placed in mainstream schools. Although these children will usually receive the support of teachers with specialised knowledge and training, more teachers without this training now share the responsibility of providing appropriate education for them. In addition there will be more than a few children in every school who experience transient hearing losses and may not become known to the specialist services. Because of the high incidence of Otitis media, the condition which most frequently causes these more temporary and reversible losses, children with other kinds of special needs may also be subject to this additional disadvantage.

Hearing impairment not only poses a threat to successful communication but can also interfere with the child's language acquisition and speech development. Often therefore, speech and language therapists are also involved with helping hearing-impaired children. In addition, they also encounter children with difficulties in speech and language development that are complicated by the additional presence of hearing difficulties, particularly of the milder kind.

It was for these reasons that we thought that this year the annual conference for teachers and therapists, hosted by the Department of Speech, would look at hearing impairment. Like other areas of special education it is an impairment with medical and educational aspects. It is important that everyone helping a child with a hearing impairment understands the concerns and responsibilities of others but this can be difficult to achieve because some are employed in health and some in education so do not have easy access to one another in the normal course of events. It seemed an excellent opportunity to bring together speakers with different concerns and backgrounds to describe recent developments and current practice so that the care and help given by each of the professionals involved is informed by this knowledge.

Chapter 1 looks at the history of provision for children with long-term, prelinguistic hearing loss in this country and at the possible effects of the recent changes in legislation on provision. Chapter 2 looks at different types of hearing loss from the point of view of the medical consultant, the factors that influence their treatment and recent developments in this field. Chapter 3 looks at the effect of different kinds and degrees of hearing loss on the social and linguistic development of children with different types and degrees of hearing loss. Chapter 4 discusses the effect of adverse acoustic settings on hearing impaired children and how these can be ameliorated. Chapter 5 considers the role of the specialist teacher in supporting and advising teachers of children in mainstream schools. Chapter 6 outlines the special skills needed by speech and language therapists who work with children with more severe and long-term hearing loss. The complexity of the subject cannot be fully addressed in five short chapters. Many of the chapters include reference to sources for further and in depth information. We have also included the addresses of organisations which may also be able to offer more specialist help and advice.

The terms 'deaf' and 'deafness' are sometimes thought to be negative terms which tend to be interpreted by the man and woman in the street as indicating complete lack of hearing. The term 'hearing impairment' is supposed to be more positive and to indicate the presence of residual hearing. For others 'deaf' is a positive identity with its own culture and language. However, throughout this book the terms hearing impairment and deafness are used interchangeably and neutrally to provide stylistic variation and reflect the preference of each writer.

Once again our sincere thanks for support in this initiative go to Sunderland Education Authority, in particular Mike Vening and Eileen Richardson; to Gillian Cavagan & Lesley Watson of the Department of Speech, Newcastle University for their secretarial assistance; and to our publishers, Mike and Marjukka Grover of Multilingual Matters.

Kay Mogford-Bevan
Jane Sadler
March 1992

Notes on Contributors

Dawn Edwards is Head of the Primary Department of the Northern Counties School for the Deaf, Newcastle upon Tyne. She is also an honorary lecturer in Education of the Deaf in the School of Education, Newcastle University. Her research interests include sign language and she interprets news headings for the local television.

Kevin P. Gibbin is a Consultant Otolaryngologist at the University Hospital, Nottingham and one of the two surgeons on the Nottingham Paediatric cochlear implant programme. He has a major interest in paediatric otolaryngology and provides support to the Children's Hearing Assessment Centre of Nottingham General Hospital.

Pauline Hughes is Head of Service for Hearing Impaired Children and Students in the Surrey County Council area. She is a teacher of the deaf and an educational audiologist and has worked in a variety of educational settings with hearing-impaired children.

Barry McCormick is Consultant Audiological Scientist and Director of the Children's Hearing Assessment Centre, Nottingham General Hospital. He has a particular interest in early detection of hearing problems and cochlear implants in young children and is author of *Screening for Hearing Impairment in Children* and Editor of *Paediatric Audiology 0 to 5 years.*

Kay Mogford-Bevan is a speech therapist and developmental psychologist and Senior Lecturer in the Department of Speech at the University of Newcastle upon Tyne. She teaches both undergraduates who are training to become speech and language therapists and experienced teachers on courses on child language and language disability. Her research interests centre on the development of communication and related abilities in children with a range of developmental disorders including hearing impairment.

Magdalene Moorey is a specialist speech and language therapist for the hearing impaired and represents the College of Speech and Language Therapists on the National Committee of Professionals in Audiology. She is particularly interested in developing communication training packages for people who support adults with communication disorders, including hearing impairment.

Jane Sadler is a teacher and speech and language therapist. She is a lecturer in the Department of Speech where she coordinates the part-time and full-time Diploma and Masters courses on Child Language and Language Disability for experienced teachers. Her research interests include teacher interaction with language disordered children.

1 Practices and Provisions for Hearing-impaired Children

DAWN EDWARDS

Historical Background

Historically the care and instruction of deaf children was catered for by the church. Rich families paid dedicated monks to live with and instruct their children and deaf children from poor families became the concern of religious groups who provided protective and training institutions for them. Early records show that in 1329 provision was made for deaf children in the first English Hospice by a hospital brotherhood. Methodism and Evangelicalism believed strongly in the salvation of the individual and these religious convictions remained a powerful impetus for the provision of education. In 1792 Henry Cox and his committee opened the Asylum for the Support and Education of the Deaf and Dumb Children of the Poor. Several of these early asylums provided by the Church have survived the course of time, becoming the non-maintained special schools which add to the provision made by local education authorities for hearing impaired children.

An example is Henry Cox's asylum which initially provided for six children but this number quickly grew to eighty and the original asylum moved to larger premises in the Old Kent Road. Ten years later there were 350 pupils in the main school together with an extensive waiting list. Consequently a branch was established in Margate where, to this day, the residential/day non-maintained special school continues to make provision for hearing impaired children. Further north, in Newcastle upon Tyne, a group of clergy, many of whom were from the Established Church in Scotland, established the Northern Asylum for the Blind, Deaf and Dumb in 1838. This also continues to make provision for hearing impaired children as Northern Counties School for the Deaf which compliments the provision made by local education authorities.

The Elementary Education Act of 1870 required School Boards to

1

provide education for all children within their district with no exceptions. Consequently many handicapped children found their way into elementary classrooms. Obvious difficulties ensued. William Stainer, Chaplain to the Deaf and Dumb, having become aware of the problem, established a separate class with five pupils in a room attached to a public elementary school in Bethnal Green. Other school boards followed this lead and over a period of ten years special classes for the deaf were established in Leeds, Nottingham, Bradford, Bristol and Leicester.

A Royal Commission was appointed subsequently by the Secretary to the Education Department, to gather information regarding the needs of deaf and blind children. The Elementary Education (Blind and Deaf Children) Act 1893 was the first legislation requiring authorities to make provision for those children from the ages of 7 yrs – 16 yrs. At last the responsibility lay squarely with school authorities to either set up a specific school of their own or to contribute towards one already providing instruction for blind or deaf children. As a result almost all diagnosed deaf children attended school on reaching their seventh birthday. Not until the Education Deaf Children's Act 1937 did legislation allow 5–7 yr olds access to the education system and this followed recommendations of the Wood Committee in the Report of 1924. (see Appendix 1.1 & 1.2).

Many legal changes were introduced over the ensuing years. School boards ceased to exist and local education authorities were formed, to be responsible for the education of children and young people in England and Wales. With the Education Act of 1944 education in this country became compulsory for non-handicapped children between the ages of five and fifteen years. This statutory system was organised into three progressive stages of primary, secondary and further education in order to meet the needs of the population within each local education authority. The Act also stipulated that parents had a legal duty to ensure that their child received suitable full-time education.

In 1945 the regulations which followed the 1944 Education Act laid down eleven categories of handicap which were clearly defined. Two of these were 'partially deaf' and 'deaf'. These two categories remained until the Education Act of 1981. Parents were required to present their child for a medical examination and the results of this determined the category of school to which the child would be sent. Schools were criticised at this time because many provided special treatment rather than special education.

As post-war classes within the state system were very large, it was often more convenient for local town authorities to establish special schools in large, country mansions or town houses.

Special education in England and Wales largely followed the legislation set out in the Education Act 1944, although several regulations were amended in the Acts of 1970 and 1976. However, significant changes were made during the 1980s. Mary Warnock chaired a committee of enquiry which reported its recommendations in 1978. The Warnock Report was considerably influential in re-examining the whole basis of special education.

It was recommended that the medical categories previously laid out were replaced by the general concept of 'special educational need'. This avoided the former requirement to classify children as handicapped or non-handicapped. The new system was designed to consider the abilities of individual children as well as their disabilities, and include temporary as well as permanent requirements. This enabled provision to cater for a wider range of problems than the medical categories of the 1944 Act.

Many in education interpreted the Warnock Report as an initiative to promote the policy of educating disabled children in mainstream schools. However, the recommendations concerning integration were rather cautious. Three types of integration were discussed: (a) locational: special units, classes or even schools were provided on the same sites as ordinary schools; (b) social integration: special classes or units sharing time and areas of the school with other children out of lesson times, such as playground, dining area, etc.; and (c) functional integration: children with special needs share lessons part-time or full-time with others. The report states:

. . . if integration is to bring all the desired benefits there must be a sufficient proportion of the activities of a school, physical, social and educational, in which a child with a disability or a significant difficulty can participate on equal terms with other children . . . (para 7.10.)

Integration was discussed in considerable detail by the committee; however, it also drew attention to the importance of special schools:

We are in no doubt whatever that special schools will continue to feature prominently on the range of provision for children with special educational needs. (para 8.1).

Although many of the recommendations in the Warnock Report did not require legislation to bring them about, the Education Act of 1981 results directly from it, and is often referred to as the 'Warnock legislation'.

The Act laid duties on LEAs to ensure that all pupils with special educational needs are identified and that these identified needs are met whenever practicable, in a mainstream school. Detailed assessment of a child's needs may, where appropriate, be undertaken by a multi-disciplinary professional group including the child's parents. Such assessment may result in the formulation of a statement of Special Educational Needs to protect the child. Such statements must be reviewed annually in consultation with the children's parents who have rights of appeal against the procedure of statement formulation and the constituent parts of the statement itself.

The Warnock Report also recommended the concept of the 'named person' who would be the single advisor from the multi-professional team and who would support the parents of children with special needs, from diagnosis to school entry and through the early settling-in to school. The Act states that the diagnosis, assessment and statementing of children relates to those resident in the LEA's area aged 2–19 years.

Often LEAs employed specialist teachers who provided peripatetic service and assumed the role of the named person for young children with early diagnosed hearing impairment.

The Education Act 1981 laid duties on LEAs and upon school governors which continue in force. The LEAs must ensure that all children identified as having special educational needs between two and 19 years have those needs met. Children under the age of two years may be formally assessed if their parents have given their approval for this to happen.

The Present

Much of what is provided today continues to be bound by the legislation of the 1981 Act. Early diagnosis and statementing of children should ensure appropriate provision is made. The child's degree of hearing loss should have a high significance in determining provision but differing philosophies and resources within each LEA will also considerably influence what is available.

Provision continues to be related to the two broad areas: mainstream schools and special schools. A hearing impaired child in a mainstream setting may be totally catered for within an ordinary class with the teacher being wholly responsible, or the teacher may have some additional specialist teaching support. A local education authority may choose to concentrate children with a similar degree of loss into a special class or unit within or attached to an ordinary school. Children with more complex or severe disabilities may require to be educated in a special school. Not all authorities support their own special school and consequently have to pay for places in day or residential special schools in another Authority to meet the special educational needs for some children.

The relatively low incidence of hearing impairment may cause small education authorities to give it a low priority and only employ one or two specialist teachers to support parents and mainstream teachers. Larger authorities can provide a fuller service which ranges from peripatetic pre-school support, primary and secondary and specialist teachers to support hearing-impaired students on further education courses. Rural areas with a wide distribution of children will also find flexibility of provision difficult. Services, therefore, can differ considerably and hearing-impaired children may be accorded different priorities in different areas as each local education authority has considerable freedom in determining what resources are necessary.

Primary and secondary schools are only able to accept hearing-impaired children if they fit into the mainstream education they already provide. Therefore there is a continuing important role for special schools in providing the special education for pupils whose needs cannot be met by mainstream education. Often these are children with multiple and severe handicaps.

In individual statements of special educational needs emphasis is laid on the type of teaching method considered suitable for each hearing-impaired child. The oral/aural method, usually associated with the mainstream education of less impaired children, stresses the use of hearing aids and amplification to make best use of residual hearing together with lipreading, for the development of speech and language. The philosophy of total communication uses a combination of sign language, speech, lipreading, reading and writing together with hearing aids and amplification. This was introduced into schools as a teaching method for more profoundly impaired children some years ago. Now bilingual education is sometimes being recommended for deaf children. This gives equal importance to British Sign Language and English within the classroom to ensure access to the curriculum and fluency as well as literacy in both languages.

The introduction of bilingual education will naturally have implications for the skills of the teacher. Good practice entails skilled language use by teachers and it may be doubtful if hearing teachers can reach a sufficient level of proficiency in sign language. There is considerable debate where sign language is used regarding the use of deaf teachers for hearing impaired children, but equally, these teachers need to be fluent in English if a truely bilingual environment is to result.

Whatever teaching method is adopted emphasis is laid on access to the curriculum. This became of greater significance than ever before with the Education Reform Act 1988 and the introduction of the National Curriculum.

The initial introduction of the National Curriculum gave clear indications that children with special educational needs had not been fully considered. Although the Act allowed for exemption of such children there was considerable pressure towards the entitlement of these children to have access to the National Curriculum. A Special Educational Needs Task Group was quickly set up and establishments providing special education were asked to provide it with relevant topics for consideration. Within the National Curriculum for example, English Attainment Target 1, Speaking and Listening there is emphasis on the ability to communicate orally and skills relating to oral communication are set out and subject to assessment. This obviously will require some modification for more profoundly hearing impaired children whose main mode of communication is sign language.

Statements of Special Educational Needs are now being framed for individual children with clear indications of the facilities, support and modifications needed in order to gain access to the National Curriculum. The introduction of statements of attainment in the foundation subjects of English, Mathematics, Science, Technology, Geography and History will clearly emphasise the stage at which the child is functioning. On the other hand it will also highlight differences between children's accomplishments. This is presenting major challenges for the teachers, although teachers of the deaf have always been involved in preparing individual learning programmes. The differentiation of attainment related to the National Curriculum may become more evident in children integrated into the ordinary class.

The Future

Political and economical uncertainties surround future developments. Already Sixth Form colleges and Further Education establishments have been taken out of the responsibility of Local Education Authorities and put under the control of Central Government. There is speculation that there will be changes in the way all educational services could be provided by central government so reducing local taxes further. This being the case we could see the gradual demise of local education authorities, at some time in the future. As previously explained there are considerable differences in LEA services for hearing-impaired children from area to areas but central government control could mean the development of a national policy regarding provision.

The Education Act 1988 makes provision for the Local Management of Schools. Such delegation of responsibility from the LEA to the schools, raises questions of whether schools, carefully managing their own resources, will wish to spend anything on making provision for hearing-impaired children in their school.

On the other hand, in October 1991, *The Children Act* came into force. This gives parents greater rights to press for the extra assistance that they consider necessary to meet the special needs of their children. Local education authorities will be under greater pressure to ensure that specialist help is available. Where the resources will come from to meet these demands appear doubtful at the moment although there are indications in the Act that the social services will have responsibility for co-ordinating help for any child who is not progressing satisfactorily.

Conclusion

Ever since educational provision for the hearing-impaired child became a statutory responsibility, hearing-impaired children have been first educated in ordinary schools then special schools and now the emphasis has moved back to mainstream schooling. Many teachers without specialist training will therefore encounter children with forms of hearing impairment. However it is clear that the concept of 'special educational need' demands the full range of provision. This is needed if satisfactory provision is to be made for hearing-impaired children with all degrees of hearing loss and to provide parental choice of educational methods and type of establishment.

Early identification and diagnosis of a hearing loss remains a priority. There is also need for family support from a sympathetic advisory teacher.

The needs of the deaf child and the choice of the parents should be the factors which decide educational placement above all else, although these are currently tempered by the availability of services in any given area.

Appendix 1.1

DIRECTIONS FOR TRAINING AND TEACHING

Deaf and Dumb Children at Home

BEFORE BEING BROUGHT TO THE INSTITUTION.

Do not indulge your deaf child, nor let him have his own way, but treat him as you do your other children.

Train him to help himself in every possible way, and always to keep himself clean and tidy.

Check and restrain his passions, correct his faults, and train him in the habits of industry.

Let the best example be set before him, as the formation of his character very much depends upon what he sees.

Be sure you treat him justly, as he cannot defend himself against the false accusation of others.

As soon as he is old enough, teach him the manual alphabet, and make yourself familiar with its use.

Teach him a few letters at a time, and make him write on a slate or paper.

Draw his attention to the common objects about the house, such as the *cat*, the *fire*, a *hat*, a *book*, &c. Write the names of these objects, and get him to spell them until they are fixed on his memory.

If you wish your child taught by the Oral Method talk to him as distinctly and as often as possible. Let him have every opportunity of seeing your face when speaking, and train him to watch carefully the movements of your lips. Words such as *Come*, *Go away*, *Sit down*, are easily distinguished, and will be readily understood: natural signs or the actions themselves will convey their meaning.

In teaching him to articulate, give him one sound at a time, and let him feel, if necessary, the vibration in your throat, nose, or head. *Papa*, *Mamma*, *Father*, *Mother*, are thus easily taught.

Do not proceed too quickly, and be sure he knows one word before he goes on with another.

The names of actions are as easily taught as the names of objects. Write such words as *walk*, *swim*, *eat*, *sleep*, &c., and imitate these actions.

Qualities, such as *hard*, *soft*, *fat*, *tall*, &c., may be taught in the same way by the use of a few natural signs.

As the intelligence of the child increases he will invent signs to express his ideas. Observe and adopt them for use in teaching him.

Teach him to write his own name and the names of his friends.

Bear in mind that it is only by very frequent repetition that success can be attained.

Do what you can (and you can do much) to develop the mind of your child. Use some effort to make him understand what is going on around him, and try to furnish him with correct ideas of natural objects—their value and use.

Moral and religious principles within a limited, but very useful degree, may also be inculcated.

Before the child is eligible for an institution for the Deaf and Dumb, send him to the ordinary district school, where he will acquire habits of discipline and a familiarity with school routine, which will be useful to him when he enters the Institution.

When he approaches the age of seven, write to the *Secretary* of the Institution, Mr. NEIL BRODIE, 26, Northumberland Street, Newcastle-upon-Tyne, and ask for a Form of Application, stating the age and sex of your child.

Appendix 1.2

Extracts from The Report for the Year 1912. Northern Counties Institution for the Education of the Deaf and Dumb

REGULATIONS RESPECTING THE ADMISSION OF CANDIDATES

1. No Candidate can be admitted as a Pupil who is under Seven or above Twelve Years of age, unless under special circumstances.

2. No Candidate shall be admitted unless he or she has been so far as can be judged, successfully vaccinated.

3. No Candidate shall be admitted who, by reason of weakness of intellect or otherwise, is incapacitated from receiving instruction. Should any child upon admission and after sufficient trial, be found incapable of receiving instruction, such child to be removed by its friends on their receiving notice to that effect.

4. The pupils will be expected to observe and they shall be subject to the rules and customs of the Institution.

Bibliography

The Education Act 1981. HMSO.

MACLURE, STUART J. 1966, *Educational Documents, England and Wales 1816 to 1963.* Chapman and Hall.

National Curriculum Council 1989, *A Curriculum for All.* Curriculum Guidance No. 2.

Prichard, D. G. 1963, *Education and the Handicapped 1760–1960.* Routledge, Kegan Paul Ltd.

Proceedings of Conference, Nottingham, November 1990. *Bilingual Education for Deaf Children From Policy to Practice.* A Laser Publication.

Warnock Committee 1978, *Special Educational Needs, Report of the Commission of Enquiry into the Education of Handicapped Children and Young People* (The Warnock Report). HMSO.

2 Medical Management of Otitis Media and Sensori-neural Hearing Loss in Children

KEVIN P. GIBBIN

Discussion of the management of children with deafness due to middle ear disease and from sensori-neural causes covers an extremely wide perspective. On the one hand sensori-neural deafness often causes a more severe or even a profound loss but fortunately presents in only a limited number of children whereas conductive deafness, typically due to otitis media with effusion, OME, produces a less severe degree of deafness but is experienced by large numbers of children. Black (1984) has raised the question of whether the treatment of this represents a modern epidemic, such is the scale of the problem. Thus, although both sensori-neural hearing disorders and middle ear pathology produce deafness, the problems the two groups of conditions present are very different and need separate consideration.

Sensori-neural deafness

Sensori-neural deafness has many different causes. It may arise from genetic disorders, diseases and other events during pregnancy, from the act of birth itself — peri-natal causes — and from infection, injury and other factors in the early years of life, meningitis being a major infective cause.

The purely medical management of the deafness caused by inner ear and/or eighth cranial nerve disorders involves screening programmes for the condition, identification of and, wherever possible, elimination of risk factors as well as the investigation, diagnosis and treatment of the hearing loss.

Prevention of sensori-neural deafness must remain the aim. In this respect, two important preventative measures have been instituted in the last

25 years: the introduction of anti-D Rhesus immunisation preventing Rhesus haemolytic disease and rubella immunisation in young women which began in 1970 in the United Kingdom.

Other infections which may cause congenital sensori-neural hearing loss include cytomegalovirus and toxoplasmosis; congenital syphilis is a rare cause but may result in serious hearing loss.

Increased awareness of the dangers of any drug exposure during pregnancy has similarly resulted in a reduction of this as a cause.

Birth trauma, prematurity and peri-natal hypoxia still present a significant group of causes of sensori-neural deafness and it may be that these various factors may act in combination to cause the deafness. A recent survey in Nottingham (Pabla *et al.*, 1991) showed that of 19 cases of sensori-neural deafness 11 were due to one or other of these causes and Newton (1985) has discussed the aetiology of bilateral sensori-neural hearing loss in some detail. Gibbin (1988) has listed the various causes of sensori-neural deafness and gives a method of grouping the various deafness syndromes.

The possibility of a genetic cause needs careful consideration if no other overt cause can be found from either history or examination. Genetic causes may be autosomal or sex-linked; the autosomal recessive types are the commonest. The importance of early diagnosis and referral for investigation and genetic counselling of the parents cannot be stressed too highly.

The whole question of screening programmes and methods of assessment and diagnosis of the hearing loss in these cases remains outside the scope of this chapter and referral should be made to the relevant chapters in McCormick (1988). Similarly, the methods of selection of appropriate hearing aids and other support often involve a multi-disciplinary team including Otologist, Audiologist, Teachers of the Deaf, Speech Therapists and others, including, of course, the child's parents.

One area where great progress has been made in recent years in the medical management of profound sensori-neural deafness is in the introduction of cochlear implantation in children. Although practised for several years in other countries in Europe, North America and Australia, it has only relatively recently been introduced into paediatric Otological practice in the United Kingdom. In 1989 the Department of Health announced funding for a limited number of centres to carry out clinical assessment of cochlear implantation in the management of sensori-neural deafness. The Paediatric Cochlear Implant Group in Nottingham received support for this initiative. To date some 18 children have received cochlear implants in Nottingham, the main indication being profound hearing loss acquired as a result of meningitis. Implantation in a limited number of children with congenital deafness is currently being carried out in order to assess the rehabilitation needs of this group. The Nottingham team uses the Nucleus Multi-Channel Intra-cochlear Device (see Figures 2.1 and 2.2).

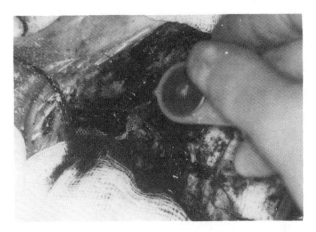

FIGURE 2.1   *A Cochlear implant being inserted.*

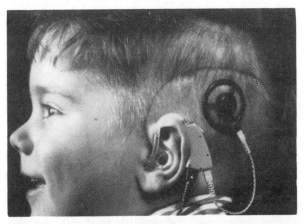

FIGURE 2.2   *A recently implanted child showing the surgical scar, the external coil and the receiver.*

Conductive Deafness due to Otitis Media

Otitis media with effusion, OME, where fluid invades the air space in the middle ear, is the single commonest cause of deafness in children and is also the commonest cause of surgical admissions to hospital in childhood. The fluid prevents the efficient conduction of sound through the chain of bones in the middle ear. Otologists are involved in all aspects of its diagnosis and treatment, being aware not only of the effects of the hearing loss on development, behaviour and education but also of the sometimes devastating effects of the underlying disease process on the middle ear and its sound conducting mechanism. Such pathology may have long-term implications and may result in the development of chronic suppurative otitis media (CSOM), that is chronic infection in the middle ear.

Glue ear, the colloquialism for OME, is widespread in children of all ages and various statistics have been presented. Brooks (1976), for example, reported an incidence of 50% in children aged 5 to 7 years. Tos *et al.* (1986) carried out a study using tympanometry and found that 60% of 150 children listed at 12 months demonstrated abnormal tympanograms, 13% with flat type B traces. Rach *et al.* (1986) showed bilateral effusions in 71% of 1,099 children examined with a marked seasonal effect.

OME may be causally related to acute suppurative otitis media (ASOM) as well as to the development of chronic suppurative otitis media (CSOM). Teele *et al.* (1980) showed an incidence of 50% by 1 year of age in a group of 2,565 children. Middle ear effusion may persist weeks or months following an episode of ASOM and may often be unsuspected. Shah (1977) found a 40% incidence of unsuspected fluid in the middle ears of 250 normal nursery school children in London.

Symptoms of Otitis Media with Effusion (OME)

The presenting symptoms of OME are varied and many cases are only picked up on routine screening. Such screening may be at the 6 to 9 month stage or at screening on school entry. It has been the author's experience that many such children are first diagnosed on behavioural testing with concomitant tympanometric evaluation following routine Health Visitor screening tests at about the age of 9 months. Were it not for such screening many of these cases might have remained undiagnosed and indeed Sade (1979) has labelled OME as 'The Silent Syndrome'. Otologists have long been aware of the many diverse ways in which OME may present and these include parental suspicion and awareness of the hearing loss, delay in speech and language development, poor school progress particularly in reading skills and behaviour problems. The latter may be attributed to day dreaming, laziness or naughtiness but in some children may include more severe problems such as enuresis, tantrums and other more marked disturbances.

Children with OME may present with mild earache, a common symptom in this condition but it should be noted that they are also prone to repeated bouts of Acute Supperative Otitis Media (ASOM). Thus, any child with recurrent ASOM should be carefully assessed for an underlying OME. A less well-recognised presentation of OME is a history of unsteadiness (poor balance) in young children in the 12 to 24 month age range. The exact mechanism of this is unclear.

There are two groups of children especially at risk from OME: those with cleft palate, where there is a mechanical impairment of the muscles acting on the Eustachian tube, which ventilates the middle ear and children with Down's Syndrome. All such children require regular otological supervision.

It is only by constant vigilance that those involved in the care of children will pick up all cases of OME and Shah (1991) has stated that the average time that elapsed between the parents' suspicion of a hearing loss and clinic referral was 16 months. The best advice to all health care and other professionals involved with children must be to heed parental doubts.

The task of diagnosis of OME is made more difficult by frequent fluctuation in the degree of deafness. Thus the audiological findings of OME may be varied. The average hearing loss is about 28 dB (Cohen & Sade, 1972) but this is not the whole story. Hall & Hill (1986) have recognised five factors which may determine the effects of the deafness in the individual child, particularly with respect to language development:

(1) The age at which the disorder occurs,
(2) The duration of the episode,
(3) The severity of the loss,
(4) Intrinsic qualities in the child,
(5) The child's environment.

In addition to the effects already mentioned, OME may produce other pathological effects on the ear which include atelectasis — collapse of the ear drum due to loss of the middle fibrous layer; adhesive otitis — fibrous adhesions within the middle ear and often a thickening of the tympanic membrane; tympano-sclerosis — a degenerative disorder with deposition of hyaline plaques in the submucosa of the ear. Tos (1981) has proposed that chronic suppurative otitis media results directly from OME in childhood and Deguine (1986) has concluded that cholesteatoma and OME have the same aetiology.

Diagnosis of OME

Clearly, diagnosis initially depends on clinical suspicion for all the reasons discussed above. Examination of the ears of a young child with an otoscope is not always easy and interpretation of all the appearances of the ear drum may be even more difficult. It may vary from seemingly normal to showing quite severe damage and it may only be by the use of the Siegle pneumatic speculum that a diagnosis may be made, demonstrating lack of drum mobility. Hearing tests administered according to the child's age and tympanometry complete the audiological aspects of the examination. However, assessment of the nose and nasopharynx are also important as chronic adenoiditis and other upper respiratory pathology may predispose to OME. This aspect will be discussed further when dealing with the treatment of OME.

One further point must be made; OME and sensori-neural deafness can and commonly do, co-exist. Thus, a child with a sensori-neural loss whose hearing deteriorates may have developed a superimposed conductive loss due to OME. Conversely, a hearing loss of 60 dB or greater in a child with OME may indicate the presence of an underlying sensori-neural deafness.

Whilst OME is the commonest cause of deafness in childhood, conductive losses may be due to other conditions of both the outer and middle ear. Developmental abnormalities of the outer ear are not uncommon and may be unilateral or bilateral. Clearly, unilateral abnormalities may excite no concern for the hearing status of the child as the other ear can be assessed and will, hopefully, show normal hearing. One of the more common causes of bilateral pinna and ear canal maldevelopment is the Treacher-Collin's Syndrome. This may occur as a chance genetic mutation or be due to an autosomal dominant pattern of inheritance. In severe cases there may be gross atresia — lack of development — of the pinna and ear canal with an associated conductive loss in the order of 60 dB.

Chronic infections in the middle ear — chronic suppurative otitis media or CSOM — may cause conductive loss. CSOM may be subdivided into two main sub-categories depending on the nature and site of the disease process.

Tubotympanic CSOM is the more common of the two types and involves infection of the mucosa — the lining of the middle ear. It is typically associated with a perforation in the main central part of the ear drum, the pars tensa and is loosely termed 'safe CSOM'.

The attico-antral form of the disease is usually associated with a defect in the attic part of the tympanic membrane and is said to be associated with a higher incidence of serious complications such as facial paralysis, meningitis and brain abscess — so-called 'unsafe' disease.

Treatment of OME

This topic remains one of the more vexed problems in Otology today. However, some general principles can be readily laid down. Glue ear is a common problem and frequently occurs in very short-lived episodes. Thus, many children need little or no treatment other than the recognition by parents, teachers and others of their temporary difficulty in hearing. Much can be achieved, therefore, by adequate and sensitive guidance and counselling of parents, reinforced with suitable written material to act as an aide-memoire. It must also be accepted that whilst it is possible to measure the individual child's hearing loss in almost all cases no two children will exhibit the same degree of disability or handicap from a given auditory threshold. Treatment will thus also depend on sensitive history taking reinforced perhaps by other tests such as the McCormick Toy Discrimination test. Such a test may also be used as a means of demonstrating to the parents their child's particular hearing difficulties, especially useful when they have not previously recognised the deafness and its secondary effects.

Medical, as opposed to surgical treatment has a minor role in the management of OME. Use of an antibiotic such as Septrin (Marks et al., 1981, 1983) has been found to be of benefit in about 30% of patients but decongestants and anti-histamines appear to have little use other than perhaps as a placebo or a form of planned prevarication.

Surgical treatment remains the mainstay of dealing with protracted periods of deafness but even here there remains the controversy as to exactly what form the surgery should take. The options may be summarised:

(1) Myringotomy and aspiration of the fluid,
(2) Myringotomy and aspiration coupled with insertion of a ventilating tube called a grommet (Figure 2.3),
(3) Adenoidectomy,
(4) Adenoidectomy plus either (1) or (2) above.

Most Otologists. are agreed that tonsillectomy has no role in the

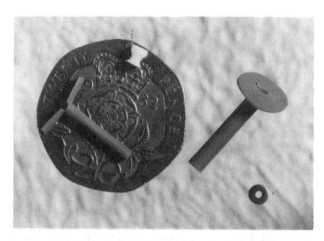

FIGURE 2.3   *A selection of different types of grommets used in the treatment of OME.*

management of glue ear and the debate centres on which combination of the listed options is the right one. Few authors address the question of relating the operation chosen to the age of the child or whether or not there is an associated adenoid enlargement or infection in deciding on the surgery. Certainly, there is little place for myringotomy alone and similarly adenoidectomy without aspiration of the fluid appears to have little merit.

It is the author's practice to carry out adenoidectomy and myringotomy in most 5 to 7 years olds, reserving grommet insertion in children in this age group for those that relapse after such treatment, approximately 1 in 5. Most other children will be treated by grommet insertion with adenoidectomy only when indicated for adenoidal symptoms.

It is a reflection on the increasing awareness and better methods of screening and diagnosis that such surgery has become increasingly common and figures from Nottingham illustrate these effects. In 1979, 71 children of 5 years and under underwent myringotomy with or without any other procedure. In 1985 the figure was 494. The rate per 1,000 ENT catchment population in 1979 was 1.75 rising in 1985 to 10.26. In case the reader feels that surgical machismo is at the heart of such a rise the figures may be compared with those of other teaching hospitals with the Trent Region of 13.30 and 13.47 in 1985.

There is wide geographical variation in the rate for this surgery at both National and International level as has been shown by Black (1985). The same author (Black, 1984) has also shown that in one Region the greatest likelihood of such surgery is found with social class I, II and III. It is this author's contention that surgical treatment should perhaps be pursued most actively in children of classes IV and V to overcome any additional social deprivation due to the deafness.

The surgery itself is usually simple and straightforward, taking only a few minutes for an experienced surgeon. Insertion of grommets is not, however, without its complications; discharge may occur but more significantly scarring of the ear drum may develop, a persistent perforation may occur and rarely cholesteatoma may develop. Typically, a Shepherd's type grommet will remain in the ear drum for 6 to 9 months before extruding spontaneously. Other types of grommet may last longer.

Much of this discussion has centred on OME and its management. The reader must remember that there are other causes of conductive deafness and these, too, may require surgery, including mastoidectomy surgery for cholesteatoma and certain other forms of chronic suppurative otitis media.

For children with bilateral atresia of the ear canal (meatus) and pinna, (Figure 2.4) until recently the options were limited to provision of a bone conductor hearing aid on a head band or a series of major ear operations with,

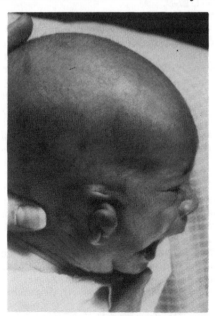

FIGURE 2.4 *A child demonstrating severe atresia of the pinna and external auditory canal.*

at best, limited success. Similarly, the cosmetic deformity of the abnormal pinna was treated surgically with only marginal benefit. The recent development of prostheses and bone conduction hearing using a bone-anchored hearing aid has changed all this dramatically. This development involves the insertion of small titanium screws into the bone on and around the ear to which can be attached a suitable prosthesis or hearing aid. Cosmetically, the results are superior to plastic surgical reconstruction of the pinna and the hearing aid is considerably superior to the conventional bone conductor device.

References

BLACK, N. 1984, Surgery for glue ear — A modern epidemic. *The Lancet* 1 (8381), 835–7.

BLACK, N. 1985, Geographical variations in use of surgery for glue ear. *Journal of the Royal Society of Medicine* 78, 641–8.

BROOKS, D. 1976, School screening for middle ear effusion. *Annals of Otology, Rhinology and Laryngology* 85 (Suppl 25), 223–9.

COHEN, D. and SADE, J. 1972, Hearing in secretory otitis. *Canadian Journal of Otolaryngology* 1(1), 27–9.

DEGUINE, C. 1986, The relationship between secretory otitis and cholesteatoma. In J. Sade (ed.) *Acute and Secretory Otitis*. Amsterdam: Kugler.

GIBBIN, K.P. 1988, Otological considerations in the first five years of life. In B. McCORMICK (ed.) *Paediatric Audiology 0–5 years*. London: Taylor and Francis.

HALL, D.M.B. and HILL, P. 1986, When does secretory otitis media affect language development? *Archives of Disease in Childhood* 61, 42–7.

MARKS, N.J., MILLS, R.F. and SHAHEEN, O.J. 1981, A controlled trial of Co-Trimoxazole therapy in serous otitis media. *Journal of Laryngology and Otology* 95, 1002–9.

MARKS, N.J., MILLS, R.F. and SHAHEEN, O.J. 1983, Co-Trimoxazole in the treatment of serous otitis media: A follow-up report. *Journal of Laryngology and Otology* 97, 213–15.

McCORMICK, B. (ed.) 1988, *Paediatric Audiology 0–5 years.* London: Taylor and Francis.

NEWTON, V.E. 1985, Aetiology of bilateral sensori-neural hearing loss in young children. *The Journal of Laryngology and Otology*. Supplement 10.

PABLA, H.S., McCORMICK, B. and GIBBIN, K.P. 1991, Retrospective study of the prevalence of bilateral sensori-neural deafness in childhood. *International Journal of Pediatric Otolaryngology* 22, 161–5.

RACH, G.H., ZEILHUIS, G.A. and VAN DEN BROEK, P. 1986, The prevalence of otitis media with effusion in two year old children in the Netherlands. In J. SADE (ed.) *Acute and Secretory Otitis Media*. Amsterdam: Kugler.

SADE, J. 1979, *Secretory Otitis Media and its Sequelae*. London: Churchill-Livingstone.

SHAH, N. 1977, Glue ears. *Developmental Medicine and Child Neurology* 19, 825–6.

SHAH, N. 1991, Otitis media and its sequelae. *Journal of the Royal Society of Medicine* 84, 581–6.

TEELE, D.W., KLEIN, J.O. and ROSNER, B.A. 1980, Epidemiology of otitis media in children. *Annals of Otology, Rhinology and Laryngology* 89, 5–6.

TOS, M. 1981, Upon the relationship between secretory otitis in childhood and chronic otitis and its sequelae in adults. *The Journal of Laryngology and Otology* 95, 1011–22.

TOS, M., STANGERUP, S.E., HVID, G., ANDREASSON, U.K. and THOMSEN, J. 1986, Epidemiology and natural history of secretary otitis. In J. Sade (ed.) *Acute and Secretory Otitis*. Amsterdam: Kugler.

3 The Implications of Hearing Impairment for Social and Language Development

KAY MOGFORD-BEVAN

Introduction

The degree to which the language and social development of a child is affected by a hearing impairment depends mostly, but not entirely, upon the type and severity of the hearing loss. Other factors, in addition to the child's intelligence, which will influence the nature of social and language development are the communication systems in use in the family, the attitude of the family to hearing impairment, the resources of the family which allow them to understand, attend to and adapt to the child's communication difficulties and any additional disabilities which the child may have.

The emphasis in this paper will be on those children with hearing impairments who are most likely to be educated within mainstream schools. Therefore the discussion will concentrate on children who have milder hearing losses since they will tend to be placed most often in ordinary classes. That is, children with mild-moderate sensori-neural hearing loss and those with fluctuating and intermittent mild conductive loss due to otitis media. In some areas of the country children with more severe problems may also sometimes be placed in mainstream schools for at least part of their education.

The Measurement of Hearing Loss

Hearing loss is usually expressed in terms of decibels (dB), the unit used to measure intensity of sound. The degree of loss is measured by the number of decibels needed to amplify a sound above the normal hearing level before it can be heard. Thus, the larger the number of decibels needed, the more severe the hearing loss.

The point at which a sound becomes audible is the hearing threshold. Hearing thresholds for pure tones can be plotted in a graphic form known as an audiogram. A pure tone used in audiometry is an electronically generated sound which can vary in pitch, or frequency, expressed in Hertz (Hz). The higher the frequency, the higher the pitch. The important range of frequencies for speech being 250 to 8000 Hz (see Figure 3.1). Vowel sounds are voiced and usually provide the loudest elements in words. Each vowel has characteristic bands of frequencies which fall towards the lower end of the range (approximately 250–3000 Hz). Consonants are generally quieter and have patterns of frequencies which include elements in the higher range (approximately 2000–6000 Hz). English fricative consonants, usually represented by the letters s, f, v, sh and ch, typically have frequencies in the upper range.

Sometimes, to give a rough indication of the severity of hearing loss, a single value is calculated from a pure-tone audiogram by averaging hearing loss across the thresholds for frequencies in the better ear. Children with a hearing loss of the same degree of severity, when measured in this way, may differ from one another in their ability to hear speech because the pattern of frequencies affected by the loss will influence how they perceive and respond to speech (see Figure 3.1 for an example).

It is sometimes hard to translate the degree of deafness measured by a pure-tone audiogram into its functional consequences. The chart (Figure 3.2) gives a rough indication of what can be expected but individual children may exceed or fall short of these expectations because factors such as motivation and auditory training can affect the use made of residual hearing. A simple explanation of audiometric techniques and tests of auditory functions can also be found in Tweedie (1987: 35–59).

Sensori-neural Hearing Loss and its Functional Consequences for Hearing

A sensori-neural hearing impairment is usually bilateral and results from a defect in the sensory receptors or auditory nerves. The severity of the hearing loss and the pattern of speech frequencies affected usually remains constant over time. A sensori-neural loss cannot normally be reversed and is most often present early in life, before language develops. Therefore, as well as impairing communication through speech such a loss inevitably interferes with the process of language acquisition.

This chapter concentrates on children described as partially hearing, or those with a mild or moderate hearing loss. Whichever of these terms is used

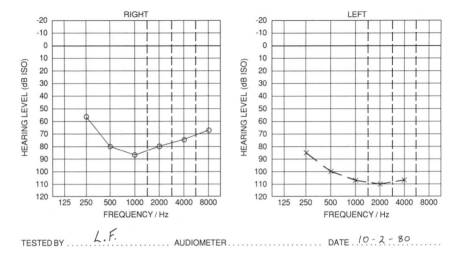

FIGURE 3.1 *This audiogram was made for a child of seven years who was attending a mainstream primary school. She has an average loss of 81dB (averaging across 500/1000/2000 Hz. in the better ear – the right) which would be classified as a severe loss. It is clear that the higher frequencies are most affected and the loss in her left ear is more severe. Her parents were both hearing and oral/aural methods were used consistently from her diagnosis at the age of four years. When seen for speech therapy at eight years she had difficulties with using high frequency fricatives, especially 's' which was often omitted in final position. This coincided with her omission of morphemes which are used in the grammar of English, for example, plurals, possessives and third person singular present verb forms. However, these relatively minor problems were overshadowed by difficulties with reading comprehension, restricted language experience and use of language forms. For example, she had difficulties in sequencing events in a narrative and using language to create imaginary events and dialogue. She attended a mainstream school at primary and secondary level until the age of fourteen. As preparation for GCSE began she requested a move to a special school because she wished to learn in the company of those with similar difficulties. In the mainstream school she used a radio aid and was supported throughout by both a speech therapist and a teacher of the deaf. Her parents took a great deal of initiative and time making this system work and excellent relations existed between all those involved. Her speech and language development were sufficient that on leaving school she obtained a job in a competitive interview with other hearing school leavers.*

it signifies that these children have some useful residual hearing. In terms of decibels, the average loss in the better ear will be between 40–70 dB. Above this level children will be regarded as having a severe hearing loss. Losses exceeding 95 dB are regarded as profound (see Figure 3.2).

For children with a moderate degree of hearing loss, a hearing aid will usually be essential but it will not always be necessary for a child to attend visually to the speaker to perceive speech. Visual attention will be necessary when precision of perception is needed, for example, when encountering new vocabulary or factual details like quantities, times or dates. Children with more severe losses will need to attend visually to spoken communication as well as using residual amplified hearing. Children with sensori-neural hearing loss can therefore be limited largely to receiving speech which is addressed directly to them so that they will miss out on opportunities to overhear the speech of others that is not directed specifically to them.

Children with a mild to moderate hearing loss are those for whom the oral/aural approach is usually recommended and is most successful. This involves training in listening with amplification so that the best use is made of residual hearing together with lip reading. However spoken language acquisition may still be delayed.

As a footnote to this section, it is worth noting that it can sometimes appear that there is an improvement in hearing in the early years. This appears on the audiograms as a result of training in listening. The child becomes more skilled in detecting and responding to sound and more attentive and co-operative in this form of testing.

Fluctuating/Intermittent Hearing Loss and its Functional Consequences for Hearing

The second group of children with hearing impairments that are most frequently encountered in mainstream settings are those with a mild and intermittent or fluctuating loss. This loss is due to a failure to conduct sound effectively across the middle ear as a result of otitis media with effusion (OME) which can be treated effectively so that it rarely becomes a long term disability. Often the loss is episodic or recurrent, associated with an acute infection though this can also be chronic.

The degree of loss is in the region between normal hearing and mild hearing loss. The average loss noted from research studies is around 30 dB though in some children it can be more severe than this. Longitudinal studies of children with this condition have estimated that episodes affecting hearing

Average loss in better ear in decibels	Degree of hearing loss	Use made of hearing for speech
−10 to 25 dB	'within normal limits'	responds to all speech in most environments
25 to 40 dB	mild loss	has difficulty responding to conversational speech especially with background noise
40 to 70 dB	moderate loss	has difficulty with all conversational speech. Perception is better with amplification and use of visual clues like lip reading.
70 to 95 dB	severe loss	difficulty with perceiving amplified speech without the aid of lip reading
95 dB and above	profound loss	although can respond to some amplified speech, what is heard carries little information of value without the use of all available visual clues.

FIGURE 3.2

last on average 30 days. Speech and language therapists and teachers may never get a satisfactory estimate of the degree of hearing loss when at its most severe because assessment is not carried out at this point. Because it is not always accompanied by symptoms which leads the child to complain, it may be difficult to decide when and for how long a child has been affected. This can make it difficult to decide what part the hearing loss has played in any speech, language or educational problems which an individual child may be experiencing.

Because the impairment is intermittent and fluctuating it is not always possible to know at any given time how much difficulty a child is having in hearing what is said. The child does not require a hearing aid but during episodes will miss quiet speech and will need to be helped by the speaker increasing their volume. The child may manage without this when the speaker is close and not competing with other sounds. The additional effort required by both speaker and listener may not be consistently maintained. Also, the effort required to attend to conversation not directed to the child may be too great to sustain all the time.

How this type of hearing loss affects the child's experience of communication can be illustrated from some parental reports of communication failure. During an episode and before treatment, for example, a child was left behind on a bus because she did not hear her mother's instructions telling her to get ready to get off over the noise of the engine. Another child was very surprised by the arrival of a relative which had been discussed at length by the family in the child's presence the previous day. Words that sound similar can be confused. One mother reported that her daughter was puzzled and disappointed when she failed to see the clowns (clouds) that were drawn to her attention in the sky. Parent's reports of children's comments after surgical treatment are also revealing. One parent told how her son asked about the noise of wind and rain which at first he found frightening. Another child was observed listening repeatedly to faint sounds which he made, like rustling tissue paper, which he had not apparently noticed before surgery.

Not only is it difficult to know the day to day hearing ability of children known to be at risk from a conductive hearing loss due to OME but not all children will have been identified.

Developmental and Psychological Implications

Describing the effects of these hearing losses on development may sound unnecessarily negative, underlining the problems rather than successes. However, the aim in this chapter is to unravel some of the complex and subtle effects that hearing disability can have on the child's social and language development without the suggestion that these are inevitable. If teachers and speech and language therapists can recognise and understand the possible negative consequences then they may be able to devise more effective ways of avoiding them.

Although the effects described apply largely to the child with the persistent and more severe hearing loss, similar phenomena have also been observed in children with less severe and temporary types of loss.

Clearly there are some consequences which follow from a developmental impairment of communication, no matter what the cause of the disability. For example, children with communication disabilities typically have difficulties in making relationships and interacting with their peers. This chapter will consider those that are specific to hearing impairment.

Hearing impairment is sometimes mistakenly regarded as a simple and straightforward matter which can easily be overcome through amplifying sound so that providing a diagnosis is made early in life, there should be few additional problems for the child. It may be understood that there is a possibility of delayed speech and language development but in all other respects development is expected to be unaffected.

It is true that unlike children with specific language disabilities that we have discussed at previous conferences, hearing impairment is almost always a peripheral sensory impairment. It is assumed that the central language learning processes are intact and able to function efficiently providing language models are accessible through the senses.

However, it is not always the case that the child's difficulties are confined to acquiring language and speech and can be simply overcome by amplification of sound by a hearing aid or the restoration of normal hearing by medical intervention.

A number of factors complicate the effects of a hearing loss. The first of these is the quality of sound that the child receives through a hearing aid. This is dealt with by Barry McCormick in the following chapter. The factors discussed here are those that relate to the development of the child in broader terms. The developmental and psychological consequences of a hearing impairment will be considered because the child's approach to acquiring language can be shaped by these consequences. The hearing impaired child may approach language acquisition with a different set of experiences of the social world.

The family context of hearing-impairment

Firstly the social and linguistic context into which hearing-impaired children are born needs to be considered. The majority of children born with or acquiring a hearing loss in the early months of life have hearing parents who communicate through spoken language. As mentioned in the previous chapter, the causes of hearing loss include genetic transmission. About 10% of children with hearing impairment are born into families where one or both parents are hearing impaired. They may also have siblings who are hearing-impaired.

It does not automatically follow that hearing-impaired parents will communicate with their children through sign language. Some parents are oral communicators and choose to use oral methods with their children. There are also many combinations of oral and manual communication that can be employed. For example, spoken language may be accompanied by natural gesture or signed English. Other parents may use British Sign Language, especially where this is their first language. The decision often also depends on the parents' schooling and experiences. Where extended families have many deaf members, signing may well be the first language of the child whether they have impaired or normal hearing. The hearing status of the child is of less significance to parents in this situation since they feel relatively confident to rear the child in either case.

For the majority of hearing parents the diagnosis of a hearing impairment is very distressing. They will probably approach bringing-up the child with less confidence than parents with a hearing-impairment and they will be faced with a number of difficult decisions concerning the communication method they will employ. Their decision will reflect the attitudes, knowledge and policy of those who advise them and the facilities available in the area where they live. They may also have no previous experience of communicating with a hearing-impaired person.

Families also vary in the way that they respond to the diagnosis. Their response will depend on whether the family is already established as a unit and experienced in rearing children before the birth of the hearing impaired child. Where a child is the second in the family to be diagnosed, parents may be more knowledgeable but not necessarily phlegmatic about the diagnosis. They may well have become skilled in communicating with the hearing-impaired child and have more knowledge about hearing loss and available services.

As well as affecting parental confidence and attitudes to child rearing, the mode of communication used in the family will determine the child's exposure to his first language. Where a hearing-impaired child is born into a hearing-impaired family who communicate through sign language, language models will be accessible from the beginning. Where the child is reared in a family that communicates through speech, there will be a delay in full access to spoken language models until a diagnosis has been made and suitable amplification provided.

Delay in diagnosis

Delayed diagnosis may have several consequences. Firstly, it has been suggested, on the strength of experiments on animals and through analogy with the human visual system, that early hearing deprivation may impair the brain's capacity to respond to and recognise the sounds of speech.

Secondly, if a hearing loss of some severity and early onset is not diagnosed in the first years of life there will be a period of development where the child learns with little or no experience of sound. Although certainly this will affect the child's experience of hearing speech and language development it will also affect experience of environmental sounds which play a part in the child's growing understanding of social events.

The child whose diagnosis is delayed will not get benefit from early amplification and the child's parents may interpret the child's lack of response to their communicative approaches in other ways. While many parents suspect a hearing impairment when these responses are missing other parents may attribute the lack of response to some failing in themselves and this can shake their confidence in their child's attraction to them. This, in turn, may undermine their attempts to communicate and establish the close emotional bond with their child which is fundamental to the development of communication. Research has shown the link between successful communication and attachment formation in young, hearing impaired children (Greenberg & Marvin, 1979).

Even when a diagnosis is achieved relatively early, towards the end of the first year of life, the child's earliest development proceeds in the absence of full access to information from environmental sound. The first year is also critical because it is the period in which communication and relationships within the family are established. Successful communication and interaction can be established through non-verbal means but parents without experience of communicating with the hearing impaired often need encouragement and support and a knowledge of the child's needs to be able to adapt their approach to interaction.

The sounds that the preverbal infant hears also have an important role in helping to make the world predictable. For example, in the second half of the first year, when the child is having solid food, caregivers often notice that the hearing infant will temporarily stop crying in hunger at the sound of food preparation. The child is able to learn from experience that the sound of one event anticipates another. Similarly, the child stops crying at the sound of the approaching footsteps of the caretaker. In this way experience comes to form sequences with an integrity and meaning. The absent sound cues can contribute to an experience which makes the world seem an unpredictable and arbitrary place. People appear to behave in unexpected ways because the sounds that help to make sense of their behaviour are missing and events, linked through time by sound, loose their integrity. For a fuller account see Gregory (1976).

This view of the world as unpredictable, arbitrary and frustrating is magnified if we consider the role that the tone of adult speech plays in interpreting, mediating and attenuating the character of events to children in the period before they understand the actual words and language used. For example, parents often use the tone of their voice to communicate comfort during painful events, or give reassurance during unfamiliar happenings. Similarly, they can signal that an event is surprising but also funny and enjoyable.

Communication in hearing children begins long before the start of language comprehension and use and is at first non-verbal. However, because communication is non-verbal it does not follow that hearing impaired infants whose hearing loss has not been diagnosed will be unaffected. Although some aspects of communication are visually accessible, for example, facial expression and gesture, parents who habitually use the medium of speech for communication do not necessarily attend much to the information they give non-verbally. This information is treated as incidental and redundant with most of the message carried by the spoken form. As a result, for the hearing-impaired child, the visible parts of the message may be truncated, irrelevant or misleading. An example may make this clearer. During a research study, a mother playing with her 20 month old son, who had a severe sensori-neural hearing loss, was encouraging him to thread some circular pieces with a hole in the centre onto a plastic pole. She told him to 'Put the pieces on the pole' However, she pointed to the top of the pole only, failing to indicate the pieces and their central hole. He interpreted his Mother's message to mean that the top of the pole was especially interesting and peered closely at it, discovering a feature which disrupted his attention to his Mother and the task in hand. Other difficulties noted in interaction between hearing parents and their hearing-impaired children involve getting and holding a child's attention, particularly to objects distant from and outside the face-to-face interaction.

It is known that the two distance receptors, vision and hearing, normally complement each other in the acquisition of language. Much that the child learns about language depends on the child mapping the language he hears onto the meaning of events, exchanges and happenings with which he is familiar and understands largely through his visual sense. He can look in one direction while he listens to a speaker who is beside or behind him.

It is also known that lip movements aid speech perception in hearing children but that hearing impaired children are more dependent on this source of information. Thus, the hearing impaired child needs his visual channel to aid his hearing and cannot easily deploy the two channels separately in the way that the hearing child does. The hearing impaired child must solve the problem of sharing his visual channel between the speaker and the object of the conversation or confine his communication to events that occur directly between speakers. Hearing impaired parents are especially skilled at using the communication space to overcome these difficulties.

Communication in socialisation

It was also observed (Mogford & Gregory, 1980) that hearing parents in communicating with hearing impaired children gradually learned to use the non-verbal context to maximum effect, physically indicating at the outset objects that were to be the subject of a verbal exchange. This, however, meant that successful communication was mainly confined to objects and events in the present.

In later years, in many families, much of social training is normally accomplished with the aid of verbal means: this includes explanation which helps to soften the frustration that is inevitably engendered in social training. When language is delayed this aspect of the child's experience and development is also affected (Gregory, 1976).

Summary

There is a danger that the hearing-impaired child experiences the world as a place which is difficult to understand. Some children come to rely on visual cues to work out what is going on and anticipate what will happen next. This becomes increasingly unreliable as the children develop and their experiences extend beyond daily routine. Another consequence is that children are tied to understanding the 'here and now'. There is also a danger that the child may resign from trying to make active sense of the world and be content to use his visual sensitivity to ensure that he fits into events but without the active effort to understand and find out what is going on when the unexpected happens. This kind of withdrawal can affect attention to auditory events, especially with children with milder intermittent losses (Hasenstab, 1987). As well as affecting responses in the classroom, language learning can also be a casualty.

A common comment made by teachers and parents about a child with a hearing impairment is that he or she 'lives in a world of his own'. On the occasions when the child misreads the cues, he may be perceived as being disobedient, especially if his hearing impairment has not been recognised. These last two occurrences apply especially to children with intermittent losses.

We have not yet considered the effect on children of having limited access to language that is not directed to them. No research has looked at the effects of overhearing communication between other speakers as a source of linguistic information and social understanding. It is likely that this is a potent source of social comment, colloquial usage, world knowledge and examples of language usage.

Effects on Language Acquisition: Sensori-neural Loss

It has already been indicated that a sensori-neural loss usually results in a delay in the onset of language. As a consequence of language delay, early and later language may be taught by parents and others rather than acquired naturally through interaction. This can affect the language that is learned, how it is used and the experience of the process of language acquisition. This may have consequences for the child's attitudes to language learning and insight into the nature of language.

In a study by Gregory & Mogford (1981), it was found that the first words of a small group of children with moderate to severe sensori-neural hearing loss tended to arise from interpersonal events in face-to-face interaction rather than to consist largely of names of people and everyday objects which is more typical in hearing children. One consequence of this was that the sudden increase in the acquisition of words, typically associated with the child's insight that people and objects have labels, seemed to be missing. Language was acquired steadily but relatively slowly so that errors persisted without correction for a much longer period than is normal for hearing children. Another feature noted was that the hearing-impaired children were more advanced in understanding their world than younger hearing children who were matched by stage of language development. In early vocabulary the hearing impaired children used cognitively more advanced concepts than their language-matched hearing counterparts. For example, the hearing impaired used words to encode the attributes of objects: size, colour and temperature. This is not typical at the single word stage for hearing children.

Although it was possible to observe stages in development similar to those in younger hearing children, the features described above meant that some unusual early word combinations were recorded which, at first sight, suggested deviant language patterns. However, the process of combination was similar to that found in hearing children at the two word stage. One example, from a child with a moderate hearing loss, will illustrate this. The utterance 'Not hot hot tea' was found to be a combination of two earlier words 'Not hot' (always used together to mean safe to touch or cold) and 'hot tea' (always used together meaning tea which is usually hot and therefore dangerous). The whole utterance was used to mean that the tea, on this occasion, was cold!

According to studies of later language acquisition the most marked difficulties are found in acquiring grammatical structures. First studies were mainly descriptive. These concentrated on written language because phonological delay and difficulties reproducing accurately the phonetic characteristics of speech, found in children with more severe sensori-neural hearing loss, made spoken language difficult to understand. These early studies described the preponderance of content words and the lack of function or grammatical words. In the 1970s, methods were developed to study the acquisition of grammatical structures and researchers debated whether language acquisition was primarily delayed or deviant. Those studying children with less severe hearing impairment largely concluded that grammatical development of spoken language was delayed rather than deviant. Authors who included children with more severe hearing loss pointed to the extreme delay in the acquisition of some grammatical abilities and the difference in order in which they were acquired compared to children with normal hearing. For a detailed review see Mogford (1988).

As a result of the delay in language acquisition grammatical structures are sometimes specifically taught to hearing impaired children. This may explain a frequently noted characteristic of later language development which is the preference for certain kinds of clause structures e.g. Subject–Verb–Object.

To illustrate the nature of expressive language here is an example of spoken language in a picture description task from an 11 year old child of below average intelligence with an average hearing loss of 92 dB. A younger child with a milder loss might show similar characteristics. The child was asked to describe a series of six pictures which show a family, mother, father, two boys and their dog, going for a drive and a picnic. The pictures were shown one at a time and the child was asked to 'Tell me what's happening here' and 'Tell me more'. Some specific prompt questions were given but these are not indicated in the transcript. Although no imitations were included, it is not possible to tell when single words were ellipted responses to questions although the authors report that there were few examples of this.

Picture 1: A car stands outside a house. The father stands by the boot which is open. Mother approaches the car carrying a basket.
Child. A car. A man. Open car. Mummy. Basket. Mummy is basket.

Picture 2: The car drives away from the house with the family inside.
Child. House. In the car. Daddy. Mummy. Boy.

Picture 3. Father and younger boy play baseball in the background. Mother watches the other boy who is looking at a book. They are sitting at a picnic bench

which is laid for four people. The dog is about to pick up a ball from the ground beside the table.
Child. Dog. Picnic. Ball. Dog is play ball. Throw the ball. Boy. Book. Read the book. Mummy looking boy book.

Picture 4: The family are sitting at the picnic table eating sandwiches and drinking. The dog is eating from a bowl on the ground beside them.
Child. Bread. Drink. Drinking. They is drinking. Dog eat food.

Picture 5: In the background the father watches the bigger boy who is doing a handstand. The smaller boy is kneeling beside the picnic table with a ball in his hand with the dog watching from underneath the table. The Mother is packing away the picnic things in the basket.
Child. Boy throw ball. In the basket. Food.

Picture 6: The car is shown outside the house with the boot and the door open. The family are walking to the house. Father carries the smaller boy who is sleeping.
Child. To home. Sleeping.

Adapted from Bench & Bamford (1979: 106)

On the LARSP profile (Crystal, Fletcher & Garman, 1976) for this child, completed from a larger language sample than shown above, the most advanced grammatical structures were at stage 4 (2.6–3.0 yrs) but the largest numbers of entries were at stages 1 and 2. Clauses and phrases showed more development than at the word level. It is evident, however, that she is able to infer and encode meaning at a more advanced level than that indicated by the level of her grammatical development. This uneven development of different facets of language means that this language is not simply characteristic of a younger hearing child.

To what extent the favouring of certain structures is the consequence of teaching language and how much the consequence of impaired auditory perception is difficult to say. Studies of hearing impaired children acquiring sign language suggest that there is no difficulty with syntax as such, when the medium is perceptually accessible. Stages in sign language acquisition appear to parallel those in spoken language in both rate and pattern of acquisition. For a fuller discussion see Bellugi *et al.* (1988) and Mogford-Bevan (1992).

Another feature of the language of children with a sensori-neural hearing loss, frequently reported by teachers but rarely noted in research, is the unexpected gaps found in vocabulary and the limited range of meanings associated with words. As a result, abstract terms may be associated with very specific concrete contexts. These limitations may not be apparent, unless probed, as hearing impaired children may not be willing to ask for assistance on every occasion when language fails to make sense. A number of factors may combine to restrict the ability to acquire meanings. Difficulty with syntax may mean that the child fails to appreciate, for example, that a word like 'preserves' can be on one occasion a noun and on another a verb. At a meta-linguistic level, the child may fail to develop, without assistance, an intuitive understanding of the derivation of words. How, for example, verbs can be created from adjectives, (e.g. general/to generalise). How words with common roots (hospital/hospitable/hospitalise) are related in meaning as well as form. They also sometimes fail to appreciate that meanings can be extended by analogy and are related at higher levels of abstraction. For example, preserves can mean 'jam' (noun) and 'protect from decay' (verb). Again, this may not be a specific feature of hearing impairment but a feature of language delay coupled with limited language experience.

In addition to difficulty in spoken language, written language is also slower to develop in children with prelinguistic sensori-neural hearing loss. As a result, the child's experience of written language is curtailed as well as that of spoken language. Reading comprehension has frequently been found to be delayed. This may be considered surprising as there is no perceptual difficulty preventing access to language in print. The hearing impaired child rarely shows difficulty in spelling words which may be one aspect of language acquisition which is relatively unimpaired by hearing loss. Thus at the level of single words, print does not cause difficulty. Difficulties with reading comprehension are less surprising when syntactic difficulties are taken into account. The non-verbal context, which plays such an influential part in the hearing-impaired child's understanding of the spoken medium is also stripped away in written language so that the child's world knowledge, illustrations and word recognition carry a substantial burden in allowing the child to construct meaning from the text. Clues that may be available in the early stages of learning to read which help the child to guess at meaning are reduced as the text advances in complexity and topics become more varied and abstract.

Effects on Language Acquisition: Flutuating-conductive Loss

Sadly, in some cases, the diagnosis of a hearing impairment may only be recognised when speech and language fail to develop. In the case of children with a mild to moderate sensori-neural loss the diagnosis of a hearing loss may well explain the late onset and delayed development of speech and language. However, this is frequently not the case when an intermittent/fluctuating hearing loss due to OME is diagnosed. The evidence linking delayed speech and language to OME is at best contentious. Children with considerable delay in receptive and expressive speech and language may be found to have a mild intermittent hearing loss which is subsequently successfully treated medically.

Although slight delays in language may disappear without further intervention, it is relatively rare for more severe delays to show rapid recovery after medical treatment of the ear condition although there may be a dramatic improvement in the child's hearing and behaviour. This may lead to a better response to treatment of the language delay. There may be some initial improvement in speech and language but this is not always sustained because while contributing to language learning difficulties, the hearing loss is rarely the sole factor involved.

The reason for this is that hearing loss due to OME is common in children with other conditions that may also delay the acquisition of speech and language. In addition, children with a specific language learning difficulty may also have an intermittent hearing loss. Bishop & Edmundson (1986) are of the opinion that the high recorded incidence and co-occurence of OME and intermittent mild loss in children with specific language disorders is the product of the energetic and systematic way in which hearing is assessed and losses treated in children showing delayed speech and language development.

It is difficult to describe the effects of a mild conductive loss due to OME on language acquisition where there is no other disability because evidence is controversial and inconclusive. The reason for this is that research is fraught with methodological problems. Studies have been criticised because they have failed to establish reliably the age of onset, length and frequency of episodes of OME, failed to disentangle hearing impairment from other disadvantaging factors and establish the hearing ability of subjects at the time at which language development was assessed. Studies have varied in those aspects of speech and language studied and samples have been small which makes it difficult to draw general conclusions.

Although some early studies found an association between chronic and continuous middle-ear disease and impairments in speech and language and cognitive and school achievements a causal link has not been established. More recent and methodologically improved studies have found little or no persistence of delays which result during episodes of hearing impairment and few long term effects of any consequence. For a review of this literature see Klein & Rapin (1988).

Teachers and speech and language therapists naturally have to think about individual children who experience problems rather than about average trends. To some extent this means examining the factors involved in each case, taking into account the frequency and severity of episodes and age of onset and detection. Other disadvantaging factors also need to be taken into account. For example, the circumstances of the family, the time and energy available to give the child individual attention. Where families and teachers are aware of the hearing loss, attention can be given to what the child may miss and efforts can be made to compensate for this. This means taking advantage of good hearing phases, looking out for and correcting misperceptions, using optimal communication strategies to make sure that the child hears as much as possible. When this can be done the consequences, in the long term, need not be of great consequence.

However, unless the possible consequences of this type of hearing loss are appreciated and the presence of the loss detected, there is a risk that behavioural and education problems may be wrongly attributed to failures in the child or his family. For example, the child's family may be blamed for lack of support and attention. Difficulties can be attributed to wilful inattention on the child's part or a low level of ability. The child then has to overcome these negative judgments in addition to catching up on missed opportunities when a loss is successfully identified and medically treated. This may make it more difficult to recover from effects of hearing impairment.

The first need in preventing negative consequences is identification. Tweedie (1987) gives the following list of signs for teachers to look out for.

(1) Day-dreaming – 'living in a world of his own'.
(2) Persistent inattention.
(3) Apparent lack of interest in what is going on.
(4) Constant repetition of 'what?' or 'pardon?' when spoken to.
(5) Naughtiness. Behaviour problems can result from stress and frustration caused by poor hearing.
(6) Speech problems.
(7) Underperforming for no apparent reason.

Hasenstab (1987) noted in preschool children that in some instances children withdrew from social situations and communication with adults and children. They would participate only in activities that were low on verbal demands and avoided eye contact, physically distancing themselves from adults. Alternatively some children became attached to and maintained close contact with a particular adult. A third behavioural symptom was overactivity and restlessness.

There are, of course, other possible explanations for any of these symptoms but they do provide a set of characteristics which would help to alert teachers and speech and language therapists to identify children at risk of this type of hearing impairment.

Once a hearing loss has been identified there are measures that can be taken to offset the effects. These can be divided into those needed before and after treatment.

Before treatment

While a child is suffering from a hearing loss the teacher or speech and language therapist can help the child by: (i) taking appropriate steps to ensure medical examination and assessment, (ii) supporting and encouraging parents in seeking treatment and assessment, (iii) understanding and managing the effects of the condition and compensating for them, (iv) making sure the message gets through to the child and repeating what may have been missed.

After treatment

Although there is rarely any need for a hearing aid or training in lip reading with a mild hearing loss, there may be a need to retrain the child to listen and become auditorily alert after the loss has been medically treated. If the child is already receiving intervention for delayed language which is explained by the presence of intermittent hearing loss, progress in language development should be steady. Being aware that treatment of the hearing impairment is not the whole answer in some children is important. Parents may not then be given unrealistic expectations about the effects of the treatment of the hearing loss on subsequent development. The child may have residual difficulties that do not recover spontaneously and still require intervention. Keeping a look out for recurrence of the middle ear problem and encouraging and supporting parents in keeping follow-up medical appointments is also valuable. Teachers and therapists who are aware of the nature of the problem can also help to prevent negative labelling, giving children fresh opportunities to achieve success in areas in which they may have previously failed.

Summary

This chapter has tried to give some insight into the complex effects of hearing-impairment. Although most children encountered by speech and language therapists and teachers in mainstream schools will be those who are least affected by their impairment, understanding some of the consequences can help to solve any difficulties that arise.

Although it is important to appreciate the effects that a receptive handicap can have on language acquisition and immediate communication in the classroom, it also helps to be prepared for some of the less obvious and more pervasive consequences. Language acquisition is intimately bound up with the communicative framework in which social understanding and knowledge of the world is acquired. The child's attitude to learning, especially language learning, may be coloured by the strategies and attitudes he develops in social interaction. The effect of a hearing loss on speech perception must be understood and the methods employed to overcome these difficulties on a day-to-day basis. These are dealt with in more detail in the following chapters. However, the cumulative effects of a hearing loss should also be understood and measures taken to manage these. The effects described are not inevitable. The degree to which these effects follow from a hearing impairment will depend on the balance between advantages and disadvantages which each child encounters. If all those concerned with supporting the child in mainstream school are aware of and understand possible effects the more negative consequences can remain potential rather than actual.

References

BENCH, J. and BAMFORD, J. 1979, *Speech-hearing Tests and the Spoken Language of Hearing-impaired Children*. London: Academic Press.

BELLUGI, V., VAN HOEK, K., LILLO-MARTIN, D. and O'GRADY, L. 1988, The acquisition of syntax and space in young deaf signers. In D. BISHOP and K. MOGFORD (eds) *Language Development in Exceptional Circumstances*. Edinburgh: Churchill Livingstone.

BISHOP, D.V.M. and EDMUNDSON, A. 1986, Is otitis media a major cause of specific language impairment? *British Journal of Disorders of Communication* 21, 321–38.

CRYSTAL, D., FLETCHER, P. and GARMAN, M. 1976, *The Grammatical Analysis of Language Disability: A Procedure for Assessment and Remediation*. London: Edward Arnold.

GREENBERG, M.T. and MARVIN, R.S. 1979, Attachment in profoundly deaf preschool children. Unpublished paper. University of Washington.

GREGORY, S. 1976, *The Deaf Child and His Family*. London: George, Allen and Unwin.

GREGORY, S. and MOGFORD, K. 1981, Early language development in deaf children. In B. WOLL, J. KYLE and M. DEUCHAR (eds) *Perspectives on British Sign Language and Deafness*. London: Croom Helm.

HASENSTAB, M.S. 1987, *Language Learning and Otitis Media*. London: Taylor and Francis.

KLEIN, S. and RAPIN, I. 1988, Intermittent conductive hearing loss and language development. In D. BISHOP and K. MOGFORD (eds) *Language Development in Exceptional Circumstances*. Edinburgh: Churchill Livingstone.

MOGFORD, K.P. 1988, Oral Language acquisition in the prelinguistically deaf. In D. BISHOP and K. MOGFORD (eds) *Language Development in Exceptional Circumstances*. Edinburgh: Churchill Livingstone.

MOGFORD-BEVAN, K. 1992, Language acquisition and development with sensory impairment: Hearing impaired children. In BLANKEN, G.B., DITTMAN, J., GRIMM, H., MARSHALL, J.C. and CLAUS, W. (eds) *Linguistic Disorders and Pathologies*. Berlin: Walter de Gruyter.

MOGFORD, K. and GREGORY, S. 1980. Achieving understanding: A study of communication between mothers and their young deaf children. Unpublished paper given at the British Psychological Society, Developmental Section Annual Conference. Language, Communication and Understanding. Edinburgh.

TWEEDIE, J. 1987, *Children's Hearing Problems: Their Significance, Detection and Management*. Bristol: Wright.

4 Acoustic Considerations for Hearing-impaired Children

BARRY McCORMICK

Introduction

The last place an experienced hearing aid user would choose to wear hearing aids is in a school setting. The acoustics are just not conducive to efficient hearing aid use for a variety of reasons. The background noise level is generally high and the lack of soft finishings produces a high reverberation effect which degrades the intelligibility of speech. These and other considerations for children wearing hearing aids in mainstream classes are the focus of interest in this article.

General Concepts

To understand the effects of classroom acoustics it is necessary to have awareness of some general concepts and terminology. Most of the disturbing effects of noise arise because of high background (ambient) noise levels and sound reflection and reverberation.

Sound levels

The intensity of sound (perceived as loudness) is conventionally measured in decibels with 0 decibels (dB) representing normal hearing threshold, 40dB being a typical background noise in a quiet room, 60dB being a conversational voice level at one metre, 80dB being a shout at one metre. In a typical classroom setting the teacher's voice will often be close to or less than the background noise level. Typical classroom noise levels are given below.

Traditional Classroom   60dB(A)
Open Plan Classroom   70dB(A)

Carpeted Unit   40–45dB(A)
Gym/Dining Room   70–90dB(A)

The 'A' in brackets after the dB symbols above indicates that the noises are measured on a sound level meter with a specific response characteristic designed to duplicate the effect of the ear's selective sensitivity to different frequencies.

Given that the teacher's voice will often be between 60 and 80dB it will be appreciated that background noise is a very significant factor in school settings. A helpful concept to consider here is that of the 'signal-to-noise' ratio and this is best understood by considering the examples given below.

Signal	Noise	S/N Radio
60dB	60dB	0dB
70dB	60dB	+10dB
60dB	70dB	–10dB

The signal-to-noise ratio is not a ratio in the conventional sense but it is the arithmetic subtraction of the noise level from the signal level. Normal hearing individuals require a signal-to-noise ratio of +6dB for satisfactory communication. It is known the hearing-impaired individuals require a more favourable signal-to-noise ratio for effective communication, that is, they are more susceptible to the disturbing effects of background noise. A hearing aid will make the signal and the noise levels more intense and will not have any effect on the signal-to-noise ratio. There are subtle effects when wearing hearing aids such that the signal and the noise are not necessarily related to the external environment but appear to originate from inside the head or ears. This experience adds to the disrupting effect of background noise.

The only solution to the signal-to-noise ratio problem is to decrease the noise at source or to increase the level of the signal. Decreasing classroom noise is clearly a formidable task and alternative strategies, discussed later in this article, must be employed.

Reverberation

Sound pressure waves disperse in all directions in free open space and the sound becomes less intense in proportion to the distance from the sound source. The inverse square law applies in this situation, that is, the sound decreases in proportion to the square of the distance from the source and each doubling of distance corresponds to a reduction in the sound intensity of one quarter (which corresponds to a decrease of 6dB).

In an enclosed space, such as a classroom, sound is reflected from surfaces within the room, particularly hard surfaces, thereby conserving the energy within the room. Hard surfaces also reflect the speech signal with the result that the direct speech signal and the reflected speech signals interfere and become prolonged. The resulting 'echo' or 'reverberation' reduces the intelligibility of speech. This phenomenon is particularly pronounced in an area with many hard surfaces such as a corridor or gymnasium and in this situation the speech may be smeared so much that it becomes unintelligible at a distance. Weak and short duration sounds, for example consonants, are masked more by reverberation. The place features of consonants, (the point of contact between the articulators) which depend greatly upon high frequency cues for correct perception, are particularly adversely affected by room reverberation. The measurement known as reverberation time (RT) is used to quantify the effect. This is defined as the time required for a sound that is produced to reduce in intensity by 60dB once that sound has been switched off. Examples of typical reverberation times are given below.

Treated classroom typically 0.4 seconds
Untreated classroom typically 1.2 seconds
Speech/conference room 0.5–1 second
Piano/music room 1–1.5 seconds
Organ/orchestral music 1.5–3 seconds

It can be seen that for music a longer reverberation time is desirable and the reverberation effect enhances the appreciation of the music. For speech, however, a short reverberation time is desirable.

Manipulation of reverberation times and signal-to-noise ratios can enhance the intelligibility of speech and these factors are particularly important for hearing-impaired individuals. A high signal-to-noise ratio and a low reverberation time should be the objective. Acoustic treatment of walls and ceilings with soft, sound absorbing materials will reduce the effect of reverberation and if heavy materials are used in the construction of walls and partitions these will help to absorb external noises thereby reducing the overall level of background noise. The use of heavy glass and double-glazing with a minimum glass separation of 20cm will add additional sound insulation. The use of soft furnishings such as curtains and carpets in addition to using acoustic tiles on walls and ceilings, will help to reduce reverberation. Sadly such features are often lacking in typical classroom settings and the desired reverberation time of 0.3–0.5 seconds is rarely achieved in practice.

Acoustic Factors Relating to Children with Unilateral Hearing Impairment

It is worth mentioning in this chapter the particular difficulties faced by children with hearing impairment affecting one ear only. It is common practice not to fit hearing aids in the affected ear if the other ear is normal. Nevertheless, it is recognised that there are specific difficulties relating to speech identification and sound localisation for these children. The fitting of a hearing aid in the poor ear may exacerbate these problems because amplification of the background noise may mask speech received through the good ear.

Even though amplification in the poor ear may not be desirable on acoustic grounds, it must be accepted that the child does have a problem particularly when speech originates from the side of the poor ear. In such circumstances, the head itself forms a barrier to sound reaching the good ear. This 'head shadow' effect will cause inconvenience for a child if not positioned so that the speaker is always on the good side.

It is known that there are subtle advantages in having two ears working well and these include:

(i) *Binaural summation* When two ears receive a signal there is a summation effect at the brainstem level which effectively adds 6dB to the overall signal intensity.

(ii) *Localisation* This advantage is lost to subjects with unilateral hearing loss who experience difficulty in locating the source of sound particularly when on the poor side. This is a particular problem in a noisy classroom where it is often necessary to view the speaker to gain supplementary visual clues. If a child cannot quickly locate the speaker some of these visual clues will be missed.

(iii) *Squelch Effect* When listening in a situation of distracting background noise, individuals with normal bilateral hearing have an ability to focus their attention on a source of sound and in some way to partially suppress or squelch the effect of the background noise. This enhanced concentration effect is lost to any individual with monaural hearing.

It will be appreciated that there are rather subtle and complicated explanations for the above phenomena. Factors for consideration include the complex design of the external ear and ear canal and the way in which it receives sound from different directions, the difference in timing of arrival of signals at the ears having travelled different path lengths, and the fact that sounds of different frequency are deflected to different degrees by objects such as the head. The end result is that the child with a monaural loss will be at risk in terms of speech discrimination ability in any normal classroom setting and this factor must be acknowledged. Modern open-plan educational settings in which children are taught in groups render impractical traditional advice such as face the teacher with the good ear, and sit near to the teacher.

Solutions

Ideally all education settings for children with hearing impairment should be acoustically treated using the methods referred to above. In practice this is not possible outside the confines of special units or special schools. For children who wear hearing aids the first priority must be to provide a radio microphone system to work in conjunction with the child's hearing aids. Such systems, commonly known as radio hearing aid systems, utilise a microphone worn by the teacher which plugs into a bodyworn radio transmitter. Radio waves from the transmitter can be detected up to 200 metres away and are picked up by a radio receiver unit worn by the child, which transforms the radio signal back to an electrical signal which can then be fed directly into the child's hearing aid system. The effect of this radio transmitter and receiver system is that the teacher's voice can be heard as clearly as if the child were standing only a few centimetres away. The teacher's voice rather than the background noise becomes the dominant signal. The disadvantage of this system is that the child hears only the teacher and not other pupils in the class. If other pupils were to be heard each would have to have their own radio microphone. Because this is impractical the child may find it necessary to switch the hearing aid microphone on and use this in conjunction with the radio microphone. Unfortunately, when the child's own hearing aid microphone is switched on this will degrade the signal-to-noise ratio because the background noise as well as the speech will be amplified. Currently there is no way around this dilemma but even as it stands the radio microphone system is an excellent, and in fact essential addition for any child hearing aid user in normal school setting. It is essential that radio microphone systems are carefully matched, and set up to suit the child's hearing aid, to avoid excessive distortion. Guidance on this topic is given in a recent article by Wood, Cope & McCormick (1990).

It is essential that radio microphone users are aware of good microphone technique. If the speaker is too close to the microphone this will overload the system producing excessive distortion and if the microphone is mounted too far away, for example at waist level, the effects of background noises will be more pronounced and the speaker's voice will sound distant. The ideal distance from the speaker's mouth to the microphone is approximately 20cm.

The provision of radio microphone systems has been the subject of negotiation and debate for many years and unfortunately a large number of radio microphone systems still need to be provided by charities. These systems should really be viewed as an extension to the child's hearing aid provision and therefore it should be the health authorities responsibility to provide and maintain the systems. The reality of the situation is that most education authorities provide such systems for use in school settings but children are not permitted to take them home.

In a survey undertaken by McCormick, Bamford & Martin (1985) it was found that 25% of a total of 13,740 child hearing aid users had been provided with radio microphone systems and the providers were as follows:

Local Educational Authority	54%
National Health Service	2.7%
Parents	2.4%
Charities	34%
Others	7%

There is little evidence to suggest that the situation has changed radically in more recent years

Induction Loop Systems

An alternative to using a radio signal is to use a magnetic signal generated by a current flowing through a wire positioned around the room. In this case the teacher wears a microphone which is linked to an amplifier which in turn drives the current around the loop of wire. The child's hearing aid is switched to a magnetic coil pick-up position, often called the Telecoil or telephone position, and this coil is activated directly by the magnetic field within the room. It is possible to have the child's microphone switched on to receive acoustic signals as well as the magnetic induction signals but in the combined mode the signal-to-noise ratio will be degraded. Induction loop systems work well within small enclosures and they have been used to good effect in airports and theatres. Induction loop systems have been largely replaced by radio microphone systems in educational settings. This is because with the radio microphone systems it is possible to select different transmission frequencies and avoid overspill to other classrooms. A combination of the loop and radio microphone systems can often be found, for example, a radio microphone might be used to transmit the teacher's voice to the amplifier which drives the loop system. This way the teacher avoids having a trailing lead from the microphone to the amplifier. At the other extreme it is possible for the final link in a radio microphone system to be that of a small inductive loop rather than a wire connection between the child's receiver and the child's hearing aid. However, the latter system, known as the neck loop system, is not recommended. The system is susceptible to changes in the strength of the magnetic field according to the orientation of the child's head within the small neck loop. Direct electrical connection from the child's receiver to the child's hearing aids should always be used in preference to the neck loop.

Space does not permit further discussion of hearing aids but a general review can be found in Wood & McCormick (1990).

Conclusions

Having established the problems faced by hearing-impaired children in poor acoustic settings in schools it seems quite remarkable that some progress as well as they do. There will always be the high flyers who can cope with adverse conditions but the groups of children most at risk are those who have to work extremely hard to maintain good progress. These children are already disadvantaged by having hearing difficulties, and are further disadvantaged by adverse acoustic surroundings. It is the responsibility of personnel working within the educational service to try to understand and, where possible, remedy the problems faced by children. It is hoped that this chapter will have offered some insight.

References

MCCORMICK, B., BAMFORD, J. and MARTIN, M. 1985, *The Provision of Radio Hearing Aids for Children*. A Report from a Working Group, RNID, London.
WOOD, S., COPE, Y. and MCCORMICK, B. 1990, A guide to fitting type-2 radio hearing aid systems in direct input mode. *Journal of the British Association of Teachers of the Deaf* 14(5), 133–41.
WOOD, S. and MCCORMICK, B. 1990, Use of hearing aids in infancy. *Archives of Disease in Child* 65, 919–20.

5 The Educational Management of Hearing-impaired Children in Mainstream Schools

PAULINE HUGHES

Hearing loss in children has for a long time been recognised as a potential educational disadvantage. It has for many years been mandatory that teachers of classes of hearing-impaired children, whether in a School for the Deaf, or a Unit, have a specialist qualification. However, since the 1960s, the trend has been for more hearing-impaired children to be placed in mainstream schools, either based in a special unit for the hearing-impaired or on the ordinary roll of the school. This has been accompanied by a decrease in the numbers of schools for the deaf and concomitant increase in external support services, usually known as peripatetic services.

In Surrey, for example, there are over 800 children with varying degrees and types of educationally significant hearing loss on the caseload of the peripatetic service. Of these, approximately 80 attend Units attached to mainstream schools and 50 attend Schools for the Deaf; principally those that cater for deaf children with additional difficulties. Nearly 700' children, therefore, attend their local mainstream school. Not all of these, of course, have severe or even moderate losses. Indeed, nearly 500 of them are not hearing aid users. Nevertheless, all these children have a hearing problem that, without the awareness and support of their families and teachers, might well affect their progress through school, and therefore possibly their adult lives.

The advantages for hearing-impaired children of working and playing alongside normally hearing and speaking peers can be enormous in terms of their speech and language and social development. Working at a pace and to the standard of their hearing peers is also a challenge that can be successfully met by the great majority. A local mainstream placement means that the child can live at home and make friends locally. However, this advantage often has to be balanced against the need for on-site help from teachers of the deaf which means a daily journey to a Unit where the child is taught alongside hearing-impaired peers. The principal disadvantages of ordinary mainstream schooling can be large classes in poor acoustic conditions. However, with the appropriate technological help and support from professional colleagues, the listening environment for most children can be effectively managed.

Factors Affecting Educational Success

Whether or not an individual hearing-impaired child 'thrives' or just 'survives' in a mainstream school is often determined by people rather than places. The first group of factors concern the child and his family. Even the hearing-impaired child who has just started school has already had many experiences, good or bad, relating to his hearing loss. The same goes for his family. Very often the personality of the child and the attitudes of his family towards his deafness will be key factors in his degree of success in mainstream school. This may well be more important than the degree of hearing-impairment or any other learning difficulty. Good pre-school family support from all the professionals concerned, particularly the Teacher of the Deaf, is instrumental in preparing the child and his family. This work cannot begin of course until a diagnosis has been made. The age of the child at the onset of hearing loss and age at diagnosis are also relevant factors in determining success. Whether a child's parents are themselves hearing or deaf is also pertinent. The majority of hearing-impaired children have hearing parents. Children whose parents are also deaf may well have more positive attitudes to their deafness and a greater maturity. Teachers may need to look at the home/school communication procedures to ensure that these are appropriate for deaf parents and where necessary adapt them. For example, if home/school books are already used, this may well be sufficient, although the school may consider getting a minicom, particularly to use in case of an emergency.

The second group of factors arise from the teachers and the school itself. In my own experience, no curriculum or timetable can be planned without a knowledge of the attitudes and awareness of the class and/or subject teachers involved. A lot of preparatory work by teachers of the deaf may be required with mainstream teachers who do not regard the hearing-impaired child as their responsibility. In some schools with Units, there may be some resentment because teachers of the deaf may be seen as receiving more pay, while working with smaller groups. In these situations, the Unit teachers have to work particularly hard to make their expertise more clearly understood, while at the same time encouraging the mainstream staff to accept at least an equal responsibility for the educational progress of Unit pupils.

Both Unit and peripatetic teachers need to have systems for monitoring, evaluating and profiling for both specific aspects, such as speech and language development, and more general aspects of the National Curriculum. They need to be able to optimise listening conditions in the classroom, as well as ensuring the fullest access for each child to the content of the curriculum.

The whole school policy towards children with special needs will also have its effect on the attitudes and awareness of staff, as will the flexibility or otherwise of the school organisation. In schools with Units, for integration to be successful, there must be flexibility in, for example, accepting other adults into the classroom, accepting a Unit child into the class, other than at the beginning of the school year or allowing the child to return to the Unit at times. Making time to talk with Unit staff, especially in team teaching situations, or where non-teaching assistants are used is also necessary for successful integration.

For the peripatetic teacher, negotiating her entry into the school, and the classroom itself, often requires sensitivity, as does arranging suitable times to talk with class or subject teachers. A major difficulty in a mainstream school can be finding a suitable place to take the child, either for tutorial support, or the occasional hearing test.

For the mainstream teacher, of course, there are many internal and external pressures on their time, that often mean that the hearing-impaired child may not come very high on the list of priorities and concerns. Recent legislation and additional assessment required by the National Curriculum has made it difficult for many teachers to give all the time they would wish to hearing-impaired children. Many teachers have classes of 30+ and possibly several children with diverse special needs in their classes.

The third factor affecting success is the role of the external support services for the hearing impaired. The policy and practice in each local education service, together with parental wishes will have a great influence on children's placements and the way in which these placements are supported. Those Education Authorities who, within the terms of the 1981 Education Act, try to provide for the needs of hearing-impaired children themselves, may well have a very different population of hearing-impaired children in mainstream schools from those LEAs who allow or encourage placement at Schools for the Deaf. In the former many more profoundly deaf children, including those with additional difficulties are likely to be placed in mainstream schools or units than in the latter. Much depends on the geography of any Authority together with its ability to attract and keep suitably qualified and experienced staff. Some rural LEAs, rather than subject children to long daily journeys to units, are placing virtually all their hearing-impaired children in local mainstream schools, with a high level of support from peripatetic staff. By contrast, in urban LEAs units or resource schools are more likely to be found.

Finally, the provision of an identifiable specialist Service for the Hearing-Impaired within an Authority's Special Needs or Learning Support provision, is crucial. In some LEAs Hearing-Impaired Services have been amalgamated with services for the visually-impaired and/or physically disabled. In other places there is a worrying trend towards generic services. If the rumoured development of the abolition of County Councils becomes a reality, many support services could be disbanded.

Classroom Strategies

All the recent trends in educational philosophy and organisation have underlined the need to provide classroom teachers with strategies that will give their hearing-impaired pupils the best educational opportunities. When looking at these strategies, it is helpful to do so from the standpoint of three principal types of hearing difficulty.

The child with glue ear

This condition mainly affects infant school children but for a few it may persist in the later years. It is particularly common in the winter months. It does not cause a severe hearing loss but its greatest difficulty, from the management point of view, is the fact that the child's hearing is likely to fluctuate. In addition, the child may be prone to absence from school because of repeated ear infections, the necessity of medical review or surgery. There may be little, if any, external support available to the teacher.

It is most important that teachers should be able to recognise the signs of hearing loss. Glue ear is often associated with colds and mouth breathing, as well as changes in behaviour, either daydreaming or being disruptive.

In general terms children with glue ear will be helped by keeping background noise and reverberation within the classroom to a minimum. Creating a quiet working atmosphere is a skill that will benefit the whole class. Schools which can run to rubber tips on chairs and tables, or even carpeting, will likewise be much more stress-free. Specifically, when talking directly to a child with glue ear, it is important to first secure the child's attention by calling his name before giving information or instructions. If the hearing impaired child is at some distance away another child should be asked to relay the instruction to avoid shouting.

In infant or junior classrooms, the old 'favourable position' for the child with glue ear, or indeed any hearing difficulty, is often very difficult to achieve but the teacher should be encouraged to stay relatively stationary and close to a 'favoured' table or two when talking to the class. 'Near and clear' is the catchphrase for talking to children with glue ear.

Children with unilateral hearing loss

It is surprisingly common for a child to have one ear without any useful hearing for speech, while the other has completely normal hearing. Children with unilateral hearing loss find it difficult to hear in noise and also to locate sources of sound, so many of the strategies that are helpful for children with glue ear will be of benefit to these children.

Particular consideration should be given to their seating position in the classroom. In principle, the child should sit with the better ear towards the middle of the room. For example, the child with a good right ear should sit with his left ear nearer the wall. For group work the child should sit with his better ear towards the majority of the group.

Outside the classroom, for example during games, the teacher should remember that the child with unilateral hearing loss may not hear from a distance if his deaf ear is towards her, or he may have difficulty locating speakers, which can be crucial if he has got the ball!

Outside of school greater care needs to be taken in traffic, as the child may not be able to tell, or may misjudge the direction of traffic, unless he is trained to be particularly visually alert.

Children with hearing aids

Children who are *hearing aid users* with sensorineural hearing losses which may be severe or even profound are also likely to have the use of radio hearing aids. As outlined previously, background noise, classroom acoustics and seating positions will all need consideration. In addition, lighting, especially of the teacher's face, is more crucial for the hearing impaired child who needs to lipread. The use of technical equipment and knowledge of methods of communication by the classroom teacher is also essential. Classrooms with good overhead lightly rarely cause difficulty in lipreading, although occasionally fluorescent lights interfere with radio aids. Teachers should avoid standing with their backs to windows, as this casts their faces in shadow. Similarly, talking to the blackboard rather than the class causes great difficulty for hearing aid users, even those with radio aids.

The most common type of personal hearing aid in use is the behind-the-ear or post-aural aid. While these aids are very helpful, they do not restore normal hearing in the way that glasses do for some people with visual problems. This is mainly due to the effects of background noise, which cannot yet be effectively filtered out and of the concomitant effect of speaker-distance. If the hearing aid user is more than six feet away from the speaker he is not likely to pick up much of what is said and lipreading at a distance is also difficult.

The benefit of using radio hearing aids is that they allow the problems of background noise and speaker-distance to be reduced if they are used effectively. By wearing a radio transmitter, the teacher is transmitting her voice directly into the hearing-impaired child's ears. However, the microphone of the transmitter must be close to the teacher's mouth. Hipster microphones or transmitters on tables are worse than useless. On the other hand, it is not good practice to leave the transmitter switched on all the time and the child will need to be able to hear his own voice, plus those of other children in the class at other times. This can be particularly difficult during class discussions but a useful strategy is to use the transmitter like the conch in *'Lord of the Flies'*, that is only the person holding the transmitter may speak! Alternatively, the child can be provided with a directional microphone which can be pointed towards the speaker. In this situation, his class mates should indicate when they are about to speak and allow a second or two before speaking so the hearing-impaired child can locate them and direct the microphone.

Simple rules of thumb for using radio aids are:

(1) The teacher should accept responsibility for switching the transmitter on and off and not allow the child to switch the receiver on and off, as the hearing-impaired child may not be aware when he is being spoken to in order to switch the receiver on!

(2) The transmitter should be on when the teacher is addressing the whole class or the hearing-impaired child directly or the group containing the hearing-impaired child. For children with moderate or even severe hearing losses, it is sometimes better to switch the transmitter off when you are speaking from very nearby, to avoid the child picking up conflicting signals. The transmitter should in any case be switched off at all other times as it is not helpful for the child to hear conversation that is not related to his work, when he may need to hear his own voice and the

conversation of those working with him. It is particularly important to remember to switch off when leaving the room!

In order for a hearing-impaired child to hear his own voice or the voices of his working group when necessary, he needs to be able to switch on and off the microphones of his personal hearing aids or the environmental microphone of his radio aid, depending on which system is being used. Young children may not know at first when to do this or may not have the physical skills to use the controls. The class teacher will need to know when to advise the child to switch on or off or even to adjust the controls herself.

In schools with units all the equipment will be checked daily before the hearing-impaired child joins his class, although it is still helpful for the class teacher to be able to carry out simple checks, especially for very young children who cannot do this themselves.

In schools without units it will often be the case that there is not a teacher of the deaf or trained assistant readily available and the class teacher will need to be capable of checking and simple fault finding.

At the end of this chapter there is a list of useful books and videos which cover this topic together with classroom strategies and equipment protocols.

Methods of Communication

The method of communication recommended for an individual hearing-impaired child may also affect classroom strategies. Methods of communication for hearing-impaired children can roughly be divided into oral and manual groups. The issues involved are highly complex and still considered controversial. In practice, however, the method of communication will generally have been decided before the child starts school.

For children being taught by oral/aural methods, there is general agreement that shouting and exaggerated lip patterns make speech difficult to follow. Knowing the child well and therefore knowing his ability to understand syntax and vocabulary should ensure that the teacher is able to use appropriate language. If the child does not understand it may be sufficient to repeat or paraphrase or simplify what has been said. Failing this, a hearing friend may be more successful in explaining or demonstrating. If this strategy also fails, it should be noted so that this can be followed up later. It is important to create opportunities for the hearing-impaired child to explain or demonstrate to hearing peers so that it does not appear to the rest of the class that it is always the hearing-impaired child who is in need of help.

In addition to using the above strategies, if the hearing-impaired child uses manual methods of communication, the teacher of the deaf is likely to have or be learning signing skills. In the mainstream classroom a teacher of the deaf may be interpreting for the hearing-impaired child and speaking without using their voice. This teacher would need to think carefully about their physical position in relation to the class teacher as inevitably a lot of the hearing children will tend to look at the interpreter as well. In these situations a good rapport with the class teacher is essential.

A class teacher may be asked to have a teacher of the deaf or an interpreter present in the room. In this case it is particularly important to discuss the lesson content in advance in case signs for subject-specific vocabulary need to be identified. The class teacher will still need to be able to communicate with the hearing-impaired child if the teacher of the deaf or interpreter is absent, therefore a basic knowledge of signing would be an advantage.

Assessment and Adaptation of the Curriculum

All teachers at the moment are grappling with the implementation of the National Curriculum and in particular the arrangements for teacher assessment and SATS for children with special needs. In principle, the continuation of good practice should be sufficient to allow access to the National Curriculum for hearing-impaired children, but all those involved must be vigilant and undertake careful monitoring and evaluation. In schools with units, decisions will need to be made about where and when hearing-impaired children are assessed. In schools without units normal classroom practices and arrangements for the hearing-impaired child should be followed. As with any other child, the SATS should be discontinued if the child becomes distressed and careful note should be made of the circumstances. Where hearing-impaired children have Statements of Special Educational Need, if exemptions from SATS are felt to be necessary, then this should be on the Statement. Similarly, any modifications and/or exemptions from the National Curriculum should be specifically stated.

In Surrey, it is felt that exemptions or even modifications, will rarely be needed for statemented hearing-impaired children. Children who are correctly placed in mainstream schools should by definition be able to cope with the National Curriculum. There is enough flexibility in the range of levels, at least up to the age of ten, to make even modifications unnecessary. This applies particularly to modern foreign languages. It is a subject area that in units particularly, has traditionally been 'sacrificed' in order to provide timetable slots for unit-based teaching or tutorial support. With the advent of radio aids and examination concessions, such as live reading of taped material, there will rarely be reasons for the hearing-impaired child of normal ability to be exempted. On the contrary, at Key Stage III, the hearing-impaired child in common with his hearing peers will start the subject at Level I. It is a subject whose linguistic content is quite carefully prescribed, which can be an advantage. Most language courses use a lot of visual material and as long as special arrangements are made for tape recorded material, which would otherwise be acoustically distorted, the hearing-impaired child has the opportunity to do extremely well. The benefits of increased confidence and self-esteem should not be underestimated. At GCSE level the hearing-impaired candidate is presented with an examination paper where language should closely reflect the content of the programme of study. This does not happen in other subjects where modified papers with simplified carrier language may be needed if the pupil is not to be disadvantaged.

For those hearing-impaired candidates who need concessions in particular subjects, if they are to be enabled to demonstrate what they have learned, these can be arranged through the British Association of Teachers of the Deaf. Concessions include live reading of tape recorded material, modified carrier language in examination papers and extra time allowances.

Conclusion

The careful thought and planning and possible changes in classroom practices may at first seem daunting for an unexperienced mainstream teacher but two important points should be remembered: firstly, care taken can in fact benefit all the children in the class, and secondly, with the additional effort the hearing-impaired child is provided with a range of educational opportunities that would not have been thought possible even twenty years ago.

Further Sources of Information

Useful books

NOLAN and TUCKER 1986, *The Hearing-impaired Child and the Family*. Souvenir Press.
WEBSTER and ELLWOOD 1985, *The Hearing-impaired Child in the Ordinary School*. Croom Helm.
WEBSTER and WOOD 1989, *Special Needs in Ordinary Schools: Children with Hearing Difficulties*. Cassell.

Useful videos

Collaboration for Successful Integration. Ewing Foundation.
Listening Through Frosted Glass. In-Form Educational Services.
Developing the Spoken Language Skills of Hearing-impaired Children. Manchester
    University TV.

Booklets for teachers

IL1   *The Hearing Aid User at Primary School.*
IL2   *Children with Unilateral Hearing Loss: Notes for Teachers.*
IL3   *Children with Unilateral Hearing Loss: Notes for Parents.*
IL4   *Hearing Problems in Young Children: Advice about Hearing Loss for Nursery and
        Playgroup Leaders.*
IL5   *Conductive Hearing Loss and its Consequences for the School-aged Child.*
IL6   *Using Radio Aids.*
IL7   *The Hearing-impaired Pupil in the Secondary School.*
IL8   *The Hearing-impaired Student.*

All available from Surrey County Council HIS.

6 Speech and Language Therapy Support of the Hearing-impaired Child in an Integrated Educational Setting

MAGDALENE MOOREY

At the present time approximately 85% of hearing impaired children in Britain are being educated in integrated settings. Two sets of guidelines on the Speech and Language Therapist's professional role were published in 1991. It is worth considering what these two documents have to contribute to our understanding of working practice in integrated settings.

The first of these publications was the British Association of Teachers of the Deaf (BATOD)/College of Speech and Language Therapists (CSLT) joint *Guidelines for Co-operation Between Teachers of the Deaf and Speech Therapists*. This document was the result of two years work by a BATOD–CSLT Joint Committee and aimed to clarify the views of the two professional bodies on collaboration at national, local and individual educational establishment level.

The second document is the CSLT guidelines on good practice, *'Communicating Quality'*, which covers all aspects of professional work including training, supervision, assessment and intervention and the role and training of the specialist speech and language therapist.

These guidelines have a number of assumptions in common.

(i) Co-operation and goodwill based on mutual understanding

Co-operation has been sadly lacking in the past between the two professional groups. Parker & Wirz (1984) attribute this to a lack of understanding of each profession's skills.

(ii) Co-operation begins at local level

However thorough and well received national guidelines are, these are meaningless without growing numbers of examples of school and unit based co-operative working practice.

(iii) A team approach to assessment and management

(iv) Team members will need additional specialist skills

It is accepted by both professions that basic training alone is insufficient to meet the needs of this group of children. The remainder of this chapter will consider the skills required of the Speech and Language Therapist and examines briefly what their professional role might be.

The Specialist Speech and Language Therapist

The first post-graduate diploma in Advanced Clinical Studies — Speech Therapy for Deaf People (ACS)—was run by the Royal National Institute for the Deaf and the National Hospitals' College of Speech Sciences in 1985. The diploma course is now run by City University. To date approximately 35 therapists hold the specialist diploma but only about 25 are currently practising. It follows that the vast majority of those hearing impaired children receiving therapy are seeing being seen by non-specialist therapists. It will be some time before every Health Authority will be able to draw on the services of a specially trained speech therapist and it is therefore necessary to clarify what role the knowledge and skills of the undergraduate training and general experience allows a therapist to adopt, with additional training from short in-service training courses.

The guidelines referred to earlier assume that the speech and language therapist has 'come out of the broom cupboard' (Roulstone, 1983) and is working not solely on direct intervention but also as a consultant and transferrer of skills to parents and other professionals.

Further, effective work with hearing-impaired children demands that we use a model of communication which views levels of linguistic function as interdependent, affecting and being affected by one another. For example, a therapist would not conclude that a child was not producing the regular plural form without first checking the phonetic transcription to ensure that a held plosive or dentalisation of a final alveolar plosive was not replacing the alveolar fricative.

[bat/bats] = [bat/bat⌐t] or [bat/bat$_n$]

Similarly, a therapist would not plan a programme for introducing the question form without first checking that the child had been given every opportunity to make use of the question form in conversation. Studies by Wood *et al.* (1986) show that some conversational partners exert such control on conversation that hearing impaired children are rarely given the initiative to ask questions.

What Knowledge does the Speech and Language Therapist Need to Work with Hearing Impaired Children?

There are three areas of knowledge which are all covered to greater or lesser degrees in the undergraduate training which will be essential: hearing and hearing loss; hearing assessment and amplification; language development of deaf children.

The therapist will need an understanding of auditory function sufficient to appreciate that hearing impairment is not simply a problem of loss of sensitivity. Therapists may or may not become involved in carrying out hearing assessments of children but all will need to be able to interpret the results of such assessments. It is also necessary to be sufficiently knowledgeable about the child's amplification system to be able to gauge what benefit the child should gain from it and also what aspects of speech will still be missed. The therapist may well need to trouble shoot minor problems with hearing aids such as battery and tubing replacement, but should also be able to identify potentially larger problems which will need the attention of the 'audiologist' such as ill-fitting ear moulds, or discomfort from over-amplification etc.

Therapists should be familiar with the literature on the spoken language development of hearing impaired children and in some authorities where a bilingual education policy exists (for example as in Leeds) they may also need to be aware of the literature on sign language development and bilingualism.

Whilst all of these topics will have been covered during undergraduate training, detailed knowledge tends to be forgotten and with time becomes out dated as research in the area develops. Two useful texts which provide overviews for revisions of these field are Bamford & Saunders (1989) and Webster (1986). The first provides an excellent review of the research literature in the areas of language development and deafness and the second is particularly relevant to the primary school child.

What Clinical Skills are Necessary for Work with Hearing Impaired Children?

The hearing-impaired child may demand clinical skills in the therapist which no other client group requires to the same extent. Again, these are all skills which may have been acquired within the undergraduate course but which may not have been used for some time.

Phonetic transcription

Few therapists would claim to have maintained the high level of transcription skills that they attained in their initial training, but the hearing impaired child's speech may demand a very high level of skill if it is to be accurately transcribed. Certain features occur in transcription far more frequently than with the non-hearing impaired child, e.g. the use of silent articulations, prolongations, non-English phonemes such as clicks and implosives. There may also be disturbances to the development of the vowel system and to prosody (stress and intonation patterns). Recording and transcribing these phonetic features is less frequently required in general clinical practice. Assessing the speech production of hearing-impaired children also demands appropriate procedures which will elicit the likely errors. The RNID Speech Assessment Procedure (King, Parker & Wright, 1985) may be the procedure of choice but with adaptation and extension to the sampling, Phonological Assessment of Speech (PACS) (Grunwell, 1985) is also extremely useful.

Visual display systems

The use of systems which will accurately and reliably represent aspects of speech visually are invaluable tools to the therapist working with hearing impaired people. They do, however, represent a large financial commitment in terms of initial funding and maintenance and therapist time in becoming familiar with all aspects of the display. An individual speech and language therapist may not feel that there is sufficient demand within her caseload to justify this expenditure but it may be possible to share resources with a therapist working in voice disorder. A knowledge of these devices will enable the therapist to recommend displays which are compatible with existing computer hardware within the school or unit.

Auditory training

This may form the bulk of work undertaken with children individually. The therapist may focus on auditory discrimination of phonological contrast discrimination of contrastive prosodic features, e.g. high fall vs. mid fall nuclear tones, and contrastive placement of the nuclear tone within sentences. The therapist's skill permits holding constant those features which are not being contrasted and varying the feature which is to be noted. For example, if the therapist is wishing to establish whether a child can contrast changing vs. steady pitch, then only fundamental frequency of voice would be altered with aspects of loudness and timing being held constant.

Manual communication

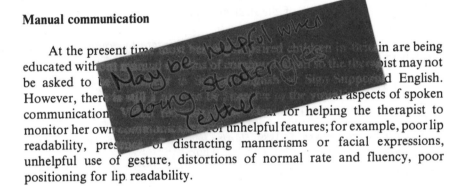

At the present tim̲e̲ ... ... in are being educated with ... ... ist may not be asked to ... ... d English. However, ther̲e̲ ... ... aspects of spoken communication ... ... for helping the therapist to monitor her own ... ... unhelpful features; for example, poor lip readability, pres̲ ... ... distracting mannerisms or facial expressions, unhelpful use of gesture, distortions of normal rate and fluency, poor positioning for lip readability.

What is the Role of the Speech and Language Therapist?

The role of the specialist speech and language therapist for hearing impaired children is clearly laid out in the BATOD-CSLT guidelines and will vary according to the nature of the educational establishment and the age of the children. The key elements however will be:

(i) Collaborative assessment with the specialist teacher.
(ii) Advice on particular aspects of communication as appropriate, e.g. class-based listening skills, social skills etc.
(iii) Assistance in planning and carrying out individual and group communication programmes.
(iv) Contributing to inservice training for specialist and mainstream teaching staff and to courses and meetings for parents.

Conclusions

Working with deaf children is a demanding and specialist field but nevertheless the skills gained during undergraduate training and general practice will allow the therapist to:

- apply knowledge of human communication to the needs of these children;
- enable the therapist as to where to gain additional information in the form of additional reading and attendance of short course such as those offered by the National Hospitals' College of Speech Sciences as precursors to the specialist training;
- deal confidently with the management of those children with intermittent and mild hearing loss who will be more familiar in paediatric experience;
- work towards closer collaborative relationships with colleagues, particularly the peripatetic teachers of the deaf and unit teachers pooling skills and resources;
- make use of the developing network of Special Interest Groups and CSLT Advisors in the regions.

References

BAMFORD, J. and SAUNDERS, E. 1989, *Hearing Impairment, Auditory Perception and Language Disability* (2nd edn). London: Whurr.

GRUNWELL, P. 1985, *Phonological Assessment of Child Speech (PACS)*. Windsor: NFER-Nelson/San Diego, CA: College-Hill Press.

Guidelines for good practice for speech therapists working with people with communication difficulties resulting from hearing loss. In *Communicating Quality* 1991. College of Speech and Language Therapists.

Guidelines for co-operation between teachers of the deaf and speech therapists (Draft) 1991. BATOD-CSLT.

KING, A.B., PARKER, A. and WRIGHT, R.D. 1985, *The Royal National Institute for the Deaf Speech Assessment Procedure*. RNID.

PARKER, A. and WIRZ, S. 1984, Towards a better understanding. *Speech Therapy in Practice*, September.

ROULSTONE, S. 1983, Out of the broom cupboard. *Special Education, Forward Trends* 10(1), 13–15.

WEBSTER, A. 1986, *Deafness, Development and Literacy*. London: Methuen.

WOOD, D., WOOD, H., GRIFFITHS, A. and HOWARTH, I. 1986, *Teaching and Talking with Deaf Children*. Chichester: John Wiley and Sons.

Addresses of Useful Organisations

British Association of Teachers of the Deaf,
Icknield High School HIU,
Riddy Lane,
Luton,
Beds. LU3 2AH.

British Deaf Association,
38 Victoria Place,
Carlisle,
Cumbria,
CA1 1HU.

College of Speech and Language Therapists,
Harold Poster House,
6 Lechmere Road,
London NW2 5BU.

National Deaf Children's Society NDCS,
45 Hereford Road,
London W2 5AH.
(Tel: 0228 48844)

NDCS Family Services Centre,
24 Wakefield Road,
Rothwell Haigh,
Leeds LS26 0SF.
(Tel: 0532 823458)

Technology Information Centre,
4 Church Street,
Edgbaston,
Birmingham,
B15 7TD.

Index